ADVANCE PRAISE

"*For over thirty years, I have been the beneficiary of Dr. Player's medical care and spiritual wisdom as my physician, dear friend, and healthcare provider to my ten thousand teammates. This book is his gift to all—clearly articulating his philosophy and demystifying the process for leading a healthier, fuller life. Reading it will be a blessing and will serve as a reference for years to come.*"

—JOE GORDER, CHAIRMAN AND CEO,
VALERO ENERGY CORPORATION

"*Thank you, David Player. I LOVE this book. Dr. Player has been my physician and friend for almost twenty years. He has walked with me through many personal trials and healthcare problems. His loving nature, medical knowledge, and expertise have been a blessing to me (and so many others). In this book, Dr. Player has instilled his great wisdom and knowledge of medicine in a way that makes complex subjects understandable. Most importantly, Dr. Player has blessed us with a resource that should encourage all of us to have an active and informed role in making better healthcare decisions.*"

—BILL TUCKER, SENIOR PASTOR, CONCORDIA
LUTHERAN CHURCH, SAN ANTONIO, TX

"For decades, Dr. Player has been liberating people with education and medical insights by asking better questions and passionately pursuing genuine well-being. In a society that has accepted sick-care for healthcare, symptom suppression instead of robust living, this book is part of his ministry of medicine, his mission to help more of us experience greater freedom and vitality!"

—MIKE SHARROW, CEO, C12 BUSINESS FORUMS

"I have known Dr. Player for over fifty years. We trained together, and later in my career, I had the benefit of working with him for seventeen years. He is the most amazing clinician I know. His knowledge of medicine is encyclopedic, and his compassion for patients is exceptional. I have often seen him resolve medical problems for patients when other providers missed the opportunity. His ability to think outside the box is his greatest skill. Dr. Player is a gifted physician who listens to patients, manages their medical issues, and provides comfort and confidence. David, I am thankful that you have shared your medical experiences in this book to help patients and physicians like me be the best that we can be."

—LAWRENCE HOBERMAN, MD, AMERICAN COLLEGE OF GASTROENTEROLOGY FELLOW, DEVELOPER OF ENDOMUNE ADVANCED PROBIOTIC PRODUCTS

"Since 1986, my family and I have enjoyed the good fortune of having Dr. Player in our lives, treating our 'whole person'—BODY, SOUL, MIND, and SPIRIT. He has guided and encouraged us to take responsibility for living healthy lives and has been a valued health coach and counselor to Lana, Benjamin, Zachary, and me. Dr. Player is a remarkable, caring, and encouraging person with exceptional medical knowledge and insight. We count ourselves extremely fortunate to have him as such an integral part of our *lives. His thoughts in this book will be a blessing for many and will encourage any who struggle with chronic health issues."*

—TOBY SUMMERS, FORMER CEO OF COCA-COLA BOTTLING COMPANY OF THE SOUTHWEST, CURRENT CEO OF MISSION ROAD MINISTRIES

"I must admit that the announcement of Dr. Player's impending retirement leaves me with a sense of nostalgia and a feeling that something great has reached its culmination. I have known, respected, relied upon, and yes, loved Dr. Player for over thirty years, and I find it sobering to think that I will not be receiving his exceptional care and annual physical exams going forward. Where will I find a physician that will pray for me and my family as part of our association? Where will I find a doctor that will sit at my feet, take off my shoes and socks and look at my feet and toes, and check my leg blood pressure and pulse? Where will I find a doctor that will speak with me about my walk with Jesus and how that positively impacts my health? Where will I find a physician that will sit with Nancy and me during my annual health review, hold our hands, and pray for us, our health, and our family? Where will I find a doctor that will give me his cell number and ask me to call him any time of the night or day if I need his assistance? These are just a few examples of the wonderful and unique friend that Dr. Player has been to Nancy and me—he cannot be replaced in my heart and mind. I pray that he will have many more years of serving our Lord and Savior, Jesus Christ, and that thousands will be helped by reading his prescription for health."

—ED KELLEY, FORMER PRESIDENT, USAA REAL ESTATE COMPANY (RET.)

"David Player has been my personal physician and friend for thirty years. Through my work with hospitals and other healthcare facilities, I have witnessed many examples of healthcare delivery. I want to say, unequivocally, that no one offers the level of care that David has given to me, to my family, and to many others. His genuine sensitivity to one's physical and emotional needs is unmatched. Many physicians allocate only a certain amount of time per patient, but not David Player. He is truly interested in each and every patient and wants to spend as much time with them as they need. He also answers phone calls, texts, and emails in a timely manner. The most important part of knowing David is that he is a deeply committed Christian. His faith is important to him, and it has been important to me as well. My visits with David always end with our holding hands while David prays for me and for my family. May God bless Dr. David Player."

—WILLIAM BALTHROPE, CEO OF MOOD:TEXAS

"I can't wait to read Dr. Dave Player's book because I know it will be a testament to his humanity, his spiritual gifts, and his skill for healing graces. I have seen Dave Player almost every year for the past twenty-one years for my executive physical—from blood work to a treadmill exercise test. Not only have I reclaimed a healthy lifestyle, but I know that David is doing God's work with every patient he sees. Each time I see Dr. Player, I'm reminded of his love of Jesus and his amazing abilities. Hanging on the wall behind his desk is a famous Nathan Greene painting of Jesus with His hand on the shoulder of the physician. I believe he is guided in everything he does by his love of Jesus and God the Father."

—SUSAN PAMERLEAU, MAJOR GENERAL, USAF
(RET.), SENIOR VICE PRESIDENT AT USAA (RET.),
BEXAR COUNTY SHERIFF (2013–2016)

HEALTH STARTS NOW

HEALTH STARTS NOW

A BACKDOOR APPROACH TO TREATING FAULTY IMMUNITY AND CHRONIC DISEASE

DAVID M. PLAYER, MD

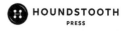

HOUNDSTOOTH
PRESS

HEALTH STARTS NOW
A Backdoor Approach to Treating Faulty Immunity and Chronic Disease

FIRST EDITION

ISBN   978-1-5445-4148-8 *Hardcover*
        978-1-5445-4147-1 *Paperback*
        978-1-5445-4146-4 *Ebook*

CONTENTS

INTRODUCTION

As I enter my fifty-fifth year of my medical career, the healthcare system as we know it has been in a perpetual state of change. A system that for more than one hundred years was based on personal relationships between healthcare providers and their patients has evolved into a complex system of telemedicine, subspecialty medicine, business and industrial medicine, modified primary care medicine (concierge medicine), and hospital-based medicine. The public has been largely unaware that these changes in healthcare were occurring. It's as if we woke from a long nap, went looking for our doctor, and found that everything had changed while we napped.

Changing technology is certainly partly responsible for the changes, but the characters in the drama have changed as well. Gone are the days of the family physician, who delivered babies, took care of three-year-olds, made hospital rounds each morning and evening, and ran to the hospital at 3:00 a.m. to see a patient who had chest pain. Those entering the world of healthcare today are often more interested in quality-of-life issues, early retirement, and accumulation of wealth than in the quality of healthcare. What begins in medical school as a philosophy of servanthood and desire to better the health of the community often morphs into chronic fatigue and dissatisfaction with a system that, for thousands of young physicians, doesn't work. It saddens me that this is the way things are.

One of the failing system's greatest fallouts is that so few physicians are involved in patients' total care. Almost everyone over age sixty has a number of physicians of various types and specialties—almost none of whom take a holistic view. There are hospital-based physicians, who see only people sufficiently ill to be in the hospital. Many are fine physicians, but to have a decent income and life quality, they work only on hospital shifts and never see lesser ill people in an outpatient office.

At the same time, various subspecialty physicians and primary care physicians never darken the door of a hospital and never, after their residencies, see anyone who is very sick. These physicians often do not know much of what is happening with their patients the instant they are ill enough to go to the hospital. Imagine the disconnect that occurs when people who were hospitalized get well and move to outpatient status to see a physician, who likely hasn't been in a hospital for years and often isn't very familiar with the important details of what goes on in hospitals. Drugs initiated in the hospital are often not the same drugs typically prescribed by outpatient physicians.

GAPS WE NEED TO BRIDGE

You may rightly ask at this point, "Why are you beginning your book, which is about the immune system, with a discussion about the failings of the healthcare system?" It's because just as there are failings in the movement of patients between inpatient and outpatient parts of the healthcare system, equal and even more important losses occur in understanding disease, due to the same processes.

Let me explain how this might occur. Those who diligently care for patients in the outpatient world are often aware of the first things that went wrong in the life of a patient—long before some severe complication of what went wrong leads to a hospital admission. Meanwhile, the hospital clinicians are often *not* aware of the behavioral problems or first symptoms that occurred when the patient was still walking about in outpatient treatment.

This disconnect causes huge pieces of interesting information to get lost between the outpatient world and the inpatient hospital world. The real cause of the disease is often long gone by the time the patient needs to go to the hospital. The man who has a heart attack did not begin having atherosclerotic heart disease on the day of his heart attack. The underlying pathology was present, slowly developing over a number of years before the big event.

This is the case for almost all illnesses, and it is why I have spent most of the last forty years or so of my medical career teaching health and wellness. As a clinical nephrologist, I've worked in both inpatient and outpatient settings for more than thirty-five years and therefore have had a better opportunity than many clinicians to gain a broad picture of the development of disease over time—as well as the life-threatening end-organ damage events that lead to death or transplantation of dead or dying organs. By the mid-1980s, I decided I could no longer in good conscience continue caring only for the dreadfully ill. I knew that, somehow, we had to move to a healthcare system that identifies serious illness far earlier than we could at that time, and do all we could to behaviorally or pharmacologically delay or prevent the development of disease. Some slight progress has been made in this regard during my years in medicine, but the abovementioned changes in the healthcare system have not been very helpful in solving the problem of evolution of serious illness, and resultant morbidity and mortality. Disease processes roll on—improved with patients' better self-care behaviors, for sure—but are often poorly understood by those in both outpatient and inpatient medicine.

My years as a nephrologist (kidney dialysis and transplant doctor) gave me opportunity to care for hundreds of different and unusual illnesses. I was able to see patients with these illnesses through months or years, watching behavior interface with genetics in incredible ways. My learning curve brought me to the brink of wanting to put down on paper some interesting things I have observed over these many years about chronic disease and its management.

But what really pushed me to begin writing was a television commercial.

THE PROBLEM BEFORE US

As I finished my workday and sat down in my easy chair, I turned on the television to listen to the news. It was not long before one of those drug company commercials came on the tube. The ad was typical of those that clutter our TV screens these days. A beautiful young woman was running through a field of grass with a dog and children trailing after her. She looked exceedingly happy—reportedly because her rheumatoid arthritis was no longer a problem since her rheumatologist was prescribing monthly "stopainimib." The commercial extolled the benefits of "stopainimib," and then began the familiar forty-five-second disclaimer:

If you receive this drug, you should check with your doctor to make sure you don't have a chronic fungal illness or TB or a malignancy, or any number of other diseases that could occur if you receive this medicine. If you experience fever, chills, sweats, joint aching, or severe weakness, you should call your doctor immediately. Common side effects of "stopainimib" include depression, recurrent infections, headache, diarrhea, rash, low blood pressure, high blood pressure, and muscle weakness. Deaths have been reported with use of "stopainimib." A rare and often fatal neurologic disease has been reported with the use of this agent.

Such ads appear on television all the time, and we are used to hearing these contrasting sides of the medicinal effects. I assume that the disclaimers are required by federal advertising laws or pharmaceutical company mandates. These ads tell us of a drug that cures symptoms of a specific disease and yet at the same time may cause illness. As I observe these commercials, I typically say to myself, "I would surely not want to take any of that stuff, since I don't want to get TB, infections, fungi, or any other terrible side effects the disclaimer declares may occur."

However, thousands of people take such medicines, and while some enjoy the benefits of their use, others suffer or even die from the drugs' side effects. Diseases for which such pharmaceutical ads are common include rheumatoid arthritis, Crohn's disease, ulcerative colitis, plaque psoriasis, psoriatic arthritis, and atopic eczema. I suspect more and more of these commercials will fill our airwaves over the coming decades, partly because the diseases being treated are becoming more common and partly because drug companies' profit margins are so great.

But what is interesting is *how* this happened. How did these treatments—with their lengthy ad disclaimers—become mainstream? I have been a physician for more than fifty years, having spent most of my career as a nephrologist, with an interest in kidney and heart transplants as well as diseases of the immune system. My experiences with a couple of thousand kidney transplants and several hundred cardiac transplants offers me a unique view of the human immune system, its function, and the ways in which drugs and human behavior may manipulate it. To effectively transplant organs, we learned we need to manipulate the immune system by suppressing it.

This same theory of manipulating the immune system is now used also to treat rheumatoid arthritis, Crohn's disease, and psoriasis. In effect, we are legitimizing the *manipulation* of the human immune system for treatment of all kinds of diseases not nearly as dreadful as a dying heart, failing kidneys, or a badly damaged liver. It's ridiculous and unsustainable. Likely hundreds of other human conditions are influenced by that dysfunction of the immune system. Are we going to continue to kill the immune system every time we treat a disease that is somehow influenced by immune activity? I'm tired of the disclaimers at the end of so many advertisements.

THE SOLUTION

I have found that the true causes of disease are often relatively simple, and can be reversed or eliminated with measures that are just as simple. Only after our ignoring or failing to try the simple approaches, over the course of months or years, complex diseases develop and require increasingly specialized physicians and other clinicians for expert care. Hundreds of diseases have been identified since I entered medicine in the late 1960s. These diseases have resulted in necessity for hundreds of specialists who care for specific diseases. The hypothesis of this book is that most diseases had very simple beginnings and could in many cases have been prevented by very simple measures. The right kind of physicians looking holistically at patients over months and years—and of course trying simple therapies—might have reversed the entire process.

What, you might ask, are these very simple beginnings? It turns out one of the greatest sources of human immune activity is in the lining of the tube that begins in the mouth and sinuses, and ends at the bottom of the bowel. It has become increasingly clear to me and others that many, if not all, of the diseases caused by disordered immunity emanate from this immune tissue that lines the sinuses and bowels. Any discussion of the immune system, and its diseases and dysfunctions, must therefore give a good idea of some things that go on along the course of the tube.

This writing is an overview, with personal stories and editorial comments, about what has led to such a change in the management of many diseases—and the television marketing to which we are all exposed. It explains how the tube might cause unknown diseases and how you, dear reader, can take better charge of your health starting now.

What I am saying is not entirely new. Good physicians have discussed these ideas for years. The problem is that the healthcare system—as it has evolved over the past fifty years—is poorly prepared to think in these ways. We must do better! It is my sincere hope that those who read this book will learn from my experiences with patients. I have certainly been blessed to be the student as well as the teacher. My prayer is that many who read this will become experts at taking charge of their own health—and taming the tube—and thus will be equipped to share these concepts with their families and friends. Perhaps they will even share them with their healthcare providers, as they seek to live long and healthy lives.

PART ONE

CHAPTER ONE

WHY AND HOW DOES OUR IMMUNE SYSTEM WORK?

Anyone who suffers from allergies understands something about the human immune system. Nasal stuffiness, runny and itchy eyes, cough, itchy ears, and a feeling of malaise are all too common symptoms for allergy sufferers. Millions of people spend millions of dollars each year when experiencing these symptoms in spring or fall—or sometimes year-round.

Indeed, over the past seventy-five years, a whole new sub-specialty of internal medicine has developed to care for the problem. Allergists and immunologists have busy medical practices in all of our great cities. They occasionally see people with severe illness, but the bread and butter of their practice is tending to people with allergic rhinitis and conjunctivitis—conditions in which the eyes are itchy and red, and the nose runs constantly, due to allergic inflammation.

All of this is to say that allergies are a common problem today—which one of us doesn't suffer or know someone who suffers from an allergic reaction? Allergies, thus, provide an excellent example of disease to help explain the human immune system's function.

HOW OUR IMMUNE SYSTEM WORKS

God created the immune system to help human beings and animals defend themselves against external invaders that might enter into or be present in their immediate environments. The immune system was created to save us from dangerous environmental chemicals or micro invaders like bacteria, viruses, yeasts, and protozoans.

Allergy symptoms such as those listed above are complex human responses to inhaled pollens, in this case viewed by the body as a toxic environmental chemical. Many people in South Texas, where I have lived and practiced medicine for more than fifty years, breathe in cedar pollen from late November through March. They experience nasal stuffiness, runny nose, itchy eyes, chronic cough, and malaise—often called cedar fever. The misery can last for months, sending people to the pharmacy or doctor's office.

The toxic environmental chemical in this case is pollen of the mountain cedar bush, which grows wild in the Texas Hill Country. When the pollen is ripe and winds blow from the north, cedar pollen content is rich in the air of South Texas. With each new breath of fresh air from the north, millions of South Texans develop related symptoms. People run to their medicine cabinets for a variety of medications designed to combat effects of the pollen invasion.

When looking into the nose, eyes, or ears of a patient who has been invaded, physicians see the classic signs of inflammation they learned the first week of medical school. The Latin names for these signs are *Rubor* (redness), *Calor* (heat), *Dolor* (pain),

Tumor (swelling), *and Functio-laesa* (loss of function). Everyone who experiences a full-blown invasion of cedar pollen knows these five signs of inflammation. They make sufferers miserable.

Interestingly, though, is that the pollen isn't creating these classic signs of inflammation—it's the immune system. Or, rather, it's the immune system's reaction to the toxic environmental chemical it considers cedar pollen to be. The pollen is not a living invader like a bacterium but simply a foreign chemical that causes inflammatory reaction in the lining membranes of the nose, eyes, ears, and sinuses.

Most amazing to me is why some people have terrible reactions to the cedar pollen and others have none at all. Some of my patients have terrible pollen allergy year after year, and use inhaled steroids and oral antihistamine medicines almost daily. Other people never suffer a single cough or sniffle during our community's cedar pollen invasion. The cedar pollen is measurable on the surface of their noses and sinuses but is not associated with any symptoms. Such people are not allergic to cedar pollen, although they may be allergic to other invaders.

Does this mean the nonallergic folks have a defective immune system that cannot respond with inflammation to the pollen invasion? Not at all. Such people may react strongly to a variety of pollens beside cedar or other environmental materials. It is also true that people who did not previously have allergic reactions to pollen can develop such allergies later in life. I have heard allergy colleagues note that it takes about seventeen years living in South Texas before a person might develop a cedar pollen allergy. This is the case with a number of my patients.

So, why do some people react to cedar pollen while others don't? And why do some people develop the allergy after several years of living in Texas while others escape? It's because each of us is immunologically unique. A unique-to-each-person antibody class known as IgE often mediates so-called allergic reactions to pollens and foods. As doctors and researchers looked at the immune system's distortions known as allergies, they discovered that many, if not all, patients with allergies had elevated blood levels of this unique class of antibodies.

What are antibodies? They are how the immune system protects us from invasions. Researchers have shown over the past seventy-five years that each human being has, when exposed to the environment, production of tiny pieces of biologically active protein known as antibodies. Of various sizes and shapes, they have the unique ability to latch on to pieces of invaders such as pollen or microorganisms. This usually results in destruction of the invader. Antibodies are made mostly in our bone marrow, lymph nodes, or specialty-type white blood cells known as plasma cells. Different types of antibodies are made in these sites, and then released into the blood and into the linings of the nose, throat, sinuses, ears, and bowels to deal with invaders or an invading substance.

IgE antibodies, with an affinity to attach themselves to cedar pollen, arrive at the lining of the throat or airway and begin the attachment process. This promotes an inflammatory reaction mediated by other white blood cells, and the area becomes swollen, hot, red, and painful. This is an example of a specific antibody mediating an immune reaction, which causes symptoms that are quite uncomfortable and might need to be manipulated with anti-inflammatory measures. This includes steroid sprays and antihistamines to blunt and inactivate the reaction the IgE antibody caused, leading to relief of symptoms.

Are there other types of immune reactions we consider to be allergies? Oh yes! Classic examples include reactions to foods mediated by IgE antibodies. Thousands of us—perhaps millions—have allergies to foods like seafood or nuts. Just as in the case of cedar pollen allergy, exposure to a food to which one has an IgE antibody reaction can be very uncomfortable and sometimes even fatal.

Chemical mediators released into the blood from a reaction between the IgE and its stimulating substance can promote release of chemicals that go all over the body and poison the lungs, blood vessels, and skin, causing low blood pressure, wheezing, cough, and severe rash. If not treated, this reaction, called anaphylaxis, can cause severe circulatory collapse and loss of life—perhaps initiated by an allergy to peanuts or shrimp, or a response to an insect sting. Countless individuals carry EpiPens and other medications designed to prevent vascular collapse in the event of an IgE-mediated allergic event.

"Allergy," then, is a negative term that describes a condition in which a normally acting immune system makes increased amounts of IgE in response to an exposure and creates undesirable symptoms. In other similarly healthy individuals, no IgE is made and no symptoms whatsoever occur despite the obvious exposure. We label one group of people as allergic or allergy sufferers, while another group with a similarly good immune system is not allergic. Doctors give medicines or injections to modify the immune responses of the first group, while the other group needs no treatment despite identical exposure to the foreign substance— be it pollen, food, insect venom, or an environmental chemical.[1]

While allergies are most commonly associated with pollen and immunological reactions, such as sneezing and coughing, the term "allergy" here refers to a wide range of reactions, and not just to pollen or food. At its most fundamental level, an

---

[1] As for those who develop allergies later in life, let's look at the cedar pollen example again. From what we know about immune system function, it would make sense that a person who was exposed over and over again might recognize the cedar pollen as foreign and develop an inflammatory reaction to it after breathing the pollen for a number of years.

allergy is *any* negative reaction to what the immune system considers a toxic and foreign invader. In such cases, the immune system is attempting to protect the body from damage but instead causes sometimes terrible outcomes more serious than sinus inflammation or a sore throat.

This, then, is the first premise of the health advice in this book:

Negative reactions mediated by the immune system are the root cause of almost all chronic human suffering and disease.

BIOFILM AND LIVE INVADERS

The second premise of this book, also revolving around the immune system, has to do with a functional part of the body most don't even know is there: biofilm.

Most immune system activity is, of course, designed to save us from live invaders like viruses, bacteria, fungi, and protozoans. The human body—both on the outer surface of the skin and all inner surfaces of our bowels, sinuses, and airways—are covered with these invaders in a layer known as biofilm. These live invaders are always with us, living outside our bodies and inside along a long passageway I call "the tube."

THE TUBE

The tube is a combination of the mouth, sinuses, upper airways, esophagus, and small and large intestines. It is about thirty-five-feet long, and its inner surface is covered with a film of bacteria and other organisms—biofilm—as shown in figure 1.

As will become apparent throughout this book, managing the tube and its microorganism inhabitants, such as bacteria and yeast, is crucial for long-term health.

35-FOOT-LONG TUBE

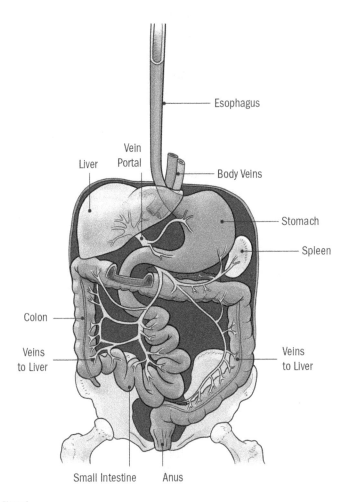

Figure 1.

But how did the tube come to be populated with the micro-organisms, or microflora?

At birth, no microorganisms were in your body, but on the way out of your mother's birth canal, you had your first exposure to your mother's bacteria. A mother's microorganisms—both bacteria and yeast—quickly colonize a newborn's bowel, and these organisms become the baby's first normal flora. The infant's immune system, very immature at this point, becomes tolerant of these organisms and begins to recognize them as normal.

Babies thus begin to develop their own antibodies against these organisms, but the antibodies formed are typically not IgE but rather other classes known as IgG, IgA, and IgM.[2] Of various sizes and shapes, these antibodies are made by white blood cells and plasma cells in the lining of the bowel, preventing microorganisms from invading the linings to enter blood circulation. A delicate balance slowly develops over the first few years of life, so that by about age three, the immune system is strong enough to protect from invaders received from the mother's birth canal and from foods other than breast milk, which is usually free of microorganisms. I should point out that breast milk contains the mother's antibodies against some of the same bacteria and yeast passed to the baby from her vaginal canal during childbirth. This is one of many reasons that babies who receive a mother's milk for months after birth are healthier and have fewer allergies later in life than infants who never received breast milk.

The immune system is well established by the third year of life and helps protect us from the invaders living in the tube over the course of a lifetime. Interestingly, as we grow older, the bowel becomes populated with an increasingly larger population of microorganisms of various sizes, shapes, and varieties

---

2   It is fortunate that most antibody-microorganism reactions are not of the IgE antibody mediated type—otherwise we would have continual allergic reactions (i.e., classic signs of inflammation in those suffering from cedar pollen allergies). The reactions are mostly mediated by IgG, IgM, and IgA antibody reactions, which are not associated with allergic reactions and their symptoms.

that do not invade but instead live peacefully along the tube linings. This is likely true not only for the bowels but also for the sinuses, ears, nasopharynx, and upper airways.

All of these surfaces are coated with a biofilm of organisms living out their existence just as we are living ours on the other side of the lining. Many of the organisms are capable of making various toxic chemicals that can kill other microorganisms—and could potentially be deadly to humans as well. The toxins typically do not kill us, however, because we have a rich immune system that sits in readiness to save us from an invasion of the living organisms and their toxins.

Sometimes, however, bad foreign invaders enter the tube, disrupting balance between the immune system and the microorganisms in the tube. This happens when a virus, bacteria, or fungus—one an individual has never experienced before—enters the scene. Salmonella, Shigella, cholera, entero-pathogenic E. coli, Candida, amoebas, malaria, and other parasites, as well as all kinds of viruses and other invaders, may enter the body and make an individual very sick. The immune system, which might not have seen any of these in the past, has to prepare to deal with the onslaught.

Sometimes the immune system is strong enough to deal with the assault. Other times, these invaders overwhelm the body's defenses and inflict heavy damage on the innermost tissues. In these cases, only antibiotics, antifungal drugs, anti-malarial agents, or antivirals might save someone's life. If one survives the invasion with use of antibiotics, antifungals, and antiviral agents, the immune system over time typically begins making antibodies and other chemicals that can deal with sub-sequent invasions from the same organisms.

To keep protecting the body from this population of biofilm and any other foreign invaders that want to join their ranks, the immune system employs not only antibodies made by white cells, called plasma cells, but also toxins made by "killer white blood cells," called lymphocytes and macrophages. These are made in the bone marrow and lymph nodes, and along the linings of the bowels and other surfaces. They form a rich layer of cellular soldiers ready to defend against any invasion of the tube linings, going to combat against the microorganisms that live on the surfaces, and in the mountains and valleys of the airways and bowels.

White blood cells and the hundreds of chemicals they make—protein chemicals like interferon, complement, antitumor necrosis factors, interleukins, and hundreds of others—are absolutely vital for survival, so much so that they deserve to be explained in proper detail. White blood cells are not really white, but since the most common cells in blood circulation contain hemoglobin, which is red, the cells containing the hemoglobin are called red cells (RBCs). Because most other cells in the blood are more neutral in color and do not contain red pigment, they are called white cells (WBCs).

There are several kinds of white blood cells, all of which are called leukocytes, and they participate with the antibodies in killing invasive microorganisms. The most important types of leukocytes in this process are polymorphonuclear cells (polys), because they have several nuclear particles within them—clearly seen when the cells are stained in the laboratory. These cells and their nuclear deposits contain enzymes that are toxic to bacteria and other microorganisms.

When a foreign invader like a bacterium or yeast tries to gain a stronghold in the sinuses, in the inner ear, or under a tooth, chemical messages, mediated by antibodies on the invaded surface, call white blood cells (polys) to come quickly to the site to deal with the invader. In very little time, a group of polys—like a pack of coyotes or wolves—arrives at the surface and kills the invader by surrounding it, engulfing it, and digesting it with enzymes in the interior of the white blood cells. This probably goes on in the lining of the lungs, sinuses, and intestines all day every day. This continued defense of the immune system is a remarkable process that goes on throughout our lives, and it is truly amazing that for at least the first forty years or so of life it works impeccably well to save most people from invasion. Antibodies reside all over the surface of the linings of the tube, and we rarely think much about the complexity of it all—at least not until we become ill.

The problem, as I've discovered, occurs when the immune system is no longer able to fight the bacteria, fungi, and germs. For most of our lives, microorganisms living in the biofilm don't usually bother us, because the immune system is so strong, and because the skin and mucous membranes are resilient and strong enough to keep out invaders. As people age, however, the skin is not the same barrier to microorganisms as it was in youth. Similarly, the inner membranes of the lungs, sinuses, and bowels change as people get older, so they do not keep microorganisms at bay as well as they once did. Therefore, an old person's immune system does not work as effectively as it did when that person was younger.

This, then, is the second premise of this book:

As we age, the immune system weakens when it comes to keeping biofilm and toxins in check—those that live in the tube and those that enter the body through the airways—possibly leading to infections with potentially serious consequences.

A COMPROMISED IMMUNE SYSTEM

Of course, such weakness of an immune system is not always caused by advanced age alone—aging is merely the most common negative factor among healthy individuals, and thus the most common cause of decreased immune system activity. But any compromise of the immune system makes one more susceptible to infection from the body's germs, as I learned early in my training.

I had been working for a couple of months as an intern at the US Air Force's largest training hospital and had not yet witnessed the death of a patient. My third rotation was to an oncology ward, where many sick patients were receiving chemotherapy. On the ward was a sixteen-year-old boy named Samuel, who had a disease called aplastic anemia caused by exposure to an antibiotic commonly used at that time. Chemotherapy was administered to destroy his native bone marrow so he could receive a bone marrow transplant from a relative. As often occurs with chemotherapy, his white blood count dropped quickly and steeply from its usual level. During staff rounds at his bed in the morning, he reported that he felt well other than a slight sore throat. His throat looked normal, and all vital signs were good. He had no fever during our rounds.

Two hours later his temperature spiked to 103 degrees, and we ordered intravenous antibiotics. Before the first dose was administered, his blood pressure dropped, and soon he was in shock. He died a few hours later of profound sepsis from the staphylococcus organisms growing on his skin and in his throat. Poisons from the staphylococcus organisms attached to his blood vessels and dilated them to a severe degree, sending Samuel into shock.

Samuel had no frontline defenses because there were no white blood cells to stand at the front door to keep invaders at bay. Without white blood cells, we had no hope of saving him—unless we had been very aggressive and presumptive by giving him the antibiotics early in the morning, when he looked well but was still brewing an infection.

It was a tragedy to lose one so young, so full of life and hope, but I learned a memorable lesson. Patients with an inadequate immune system—especially those with chemotherapy-induced white blood cell counts that are very low—are vulnerable to swift death from exposure to their own germs. We all walk around in a world full of germs and rarely become ill, because our immune systems—including white blood cells, antibodies, and a ton of immune chemicals—are doing surveillance and saving us from the germs that live in and around us. When that immune system stops working due to age or because it is otherwise compromised, the results are often deadly.

WHAT'S NEXT?

Both main premises of this book revolve around the immune system—either its reaction that is meant to protect us but instead causes more damage, or its failure due to age to defend from microorganisms in the tube and in the environment that led to harmful infections. The book overall is dedicated to unpacking these premises and navigating how I arrived at my conclusions, how they fit in with the medical community's accepted wisdom, and how you, dear reader, can take powerful control of your personal health and treatment options.

The immune system remains far more complex than any of us can fully understand. We have learned much about it over the past one hundred years or so, but what we know is still dwarfed by what we do not know—and that keeps us open to new ideas and thinking outside the box. The following chapters explore the immune system through two lenses: blood typing and organ transplantation. These are two ways in which the medical community began to better understand how the immune system is configured and just how intricate it truly is.

CHAPTER TWO

———

THROUGH THE LENS OF BLOOD TYPING

The very first revelation on how the immune system works occurred during the first attempts at blood transfusion. The first routine transplants were done in European battlefields during World War I.[3] Very early, it was learned that when type A blood is transfused into a person with type O blood, the donor blood cells are immediately destroyed, blood pressure drops, fever develops, and the recipient of the mismatched blood can develop a severe allergic reaction with trouble breathing, skin rash, and severe malaise.

What causes this terrible event? Individuals with type O blood have preformed antibodies in their blood—antibodies directed against the red blood cells of a person with type A or type B blood. Transfusion of type A or type B blood into a person with type O blood therefore causes a terrible medical

———

3   The first blood transfusion was done much earlier than World War I, in 1667 with sheep's blood transfused into a young boy who was bleeding. During World War I, however, citrate availability allowed blood to be stored and used on the battlefield, so transplants became more routine.

event called transfusion reaction, which can possibly cause the recipient's loss of life. This is, of course, the reason we have blood banks, which routinely screen all donated blood for basic type.

BLOOD TYPES AND COMPLICATIONS

In North America, we typically see people with type A, type B, type O, or type AB blood. Type A has antibodies against type B, but not against type O. Type B has antibodies against type A, but not against type O. Type AB has no preformed antibodies against any of the other types. Type O has antibodies against all the others. Interestingly, type O lacks some identifying surface proteins of A and B. People with type O can, therefore, donate blood to anybody, without risk of a transfusion reaction occurring. This is why people with type O are called universal donors. Those with type AB can receive blood from any others, without risk of a transfusion reaction occurring. They are referred to as universal receivers.

Adverse reactions to transfused blood were the first clinically important events that allowed us to observe the uniqueness of the immune system. For a long time, it seemed all human beings functioned in much the same way, but attempts to transfuse blood proved our immune systems are very unique and that unmatched blood transfusions can lead to serious medical complications.

Indeed, there is much complexity to blood typing that goes far beyond types A, B, AB, or O. Not only are there racially specific types of hemoglobin, such as type S (in patients with sickle cell disease) and hemoglobin C (a rare abnormality seen most often in African-Americans), but there are also other proteins on the surface of red blood cells that influence the immune system. The most notable and worthy of discussion are those related to the Rh system.

Patients are said to be Rh-positive or Rh-negative, depending on whether or not their red blood cells contain the Rh protein on their surface. Blood banks routinely do typing for this factor, because transfusion of Rh-positive blood into a recipient who does not have this factor can result in a rather severe transfusion reaction.

This is most important in gynecology, since a mother who is Rh-negative (lacks the Rh protein) may after her first pregnancy become exposed to the blood of her Rh-positive baby during the birth process and thereafter develop antibodies against the Rh protein. This has no effect whatsoever on the newborn, and the mother would not be aware she had become sensitized or immunologically turned on to her baby's blood. If her second pregnancy, however, were to result in an infant who is Rh-positive like its older sibling, the mother's antibodies against the Rh factor would begin to cause a transfusion reaction in the baby—even in the uterus throughout the pregnancy.

The transfusion reaction would then result in a baby who is yellow at birth because of the color of blood that has undergone the breakdown of red cells. This loss of integrity of the lining of the red blood cells is known as hemolysis. With each subsequent pregnancy, if the baby is Rh-positive (from an Rh-positive father), the transfusion reaction is expected to worsen, and it becomes more likely the child will be stillborn or severely debilitated from the intrauterine transfusion reaction.

Since the late 1960s, obstetricians have had in their offices a wonderful medicine called RhoGAM, which is essentially an antibody against the mother's antibody to Rh factor. If given immediately after a first pregnancy, RhoGAM cancels the mother's capability of making antibodies against her first baby's Rh factor-positive red blood cells. This then makes it possible for the mother to enter into another pregnancy without risk of killing her subsequent children's red blood cells.

This phenomenon turned out to be especially important in my family. My wife, Beth, has Rh-negative blood. We found out during her first pregnancy, with our daughter Amy. Because I was Rh-positive, Amy was Rh-positive as well. Thankfully, RhoGAM, which was not commercially available at that time, was made available to my family, and Beth received a dosage of this wonderful "immune antibody medicine" at the time of our daughter's birth. Two years later, our second daughter, Heidi, was born and was, as expected, Rh-positive like her father. Again, Beth received RhoGAM, which was now commercially available. The same process occurred during Beth's subsequent pregnancies with our sons, John Nathaniel (Nat) and Daniel.

I know in my heart that had RhoGAM been unavailable at the time of Amy's birth, Heidi would have been quite ill at her birth. Nat and Daniel likely would never have made it to a healthy birth. What a blessing this immune system breakthrough was for our family.

Clearly, the immune system is very complex—likely far more so than we know at the time of this writing. Blood types clearly are a consequence of immunity, determining what the body will accept or reject. Over the years, physicians have argued that this extends not only to what blood can be transfused into our veins, but also to what our bodies will allow us to eat.

BLOOD TYPES AND FOOD

Not surprisingly, over time some physicians and nutritionists have made other interesting observations related to various blood types and overall health. We know assuredly that transfusion reactions are caused by antibodies directed against protein structures on the walls of red blood cells. During the coronavirus pandemic, many physicians noted that patients with type O blood seemed to have stronger immunity against the coronavirus than did patients with other blood types. The reasons for this are unknown, but immunity to viruses and other microorganisms must have some blood type uniqueness.

Similarly, other clinicians have in the last half century suggested that some individuals with type O blood, for instance, have low-grade antibody reactions against various foods, while patients with type A blood seem to have similar reactions against very different foods. The same seems to exist for blood types AB and B. In other words, the entire immune system makeup seems to be different for people of different blood types, and some disease symptoms may be related to this phenomenon.

It's important to note that the antibodies to foods are not IgE antibodies like those present in the blood of allergy patients. People with IgE antibodies to foods may have severe symptoms with a food exposure and develop hives, wheezing, low blood pressure, and even death from cardiovascular collapse. In such cases, the allergy is obvious and the immune reaction swift and often deadly.

But the antibodies to foods in some individuals of different blood types are of a different class called IgG. These are more like the antibodies made against viruses, bacteria, and other microorganisms. Allergists acknowledge that many people have such antibodies existing in their blood. Nevertheless, most allergists do not believe such antibodies cause negative symptoms or diseases. The reason for this is that these IgG food antibodies do not cause severe allergic symptoms like those experienced with exposure to certain foods, such as IgE antibodies against nuts or shrimp in susceptible individuals.

Symptoms in patients with IgG antibodies to foods are more subtle and chronic.

A number of clinicians who have written about food sensitivities argue that the lack of immediacy of the IgG reaction makes it no less important than the IgE reaction—it just makes it more difficult to detect. When someone has IgG antibodies to a certain food and eats that food, the individual does not experience immediate symptoms from the sensitivity. Instead of developing a rash, facial swelling, or trouble breathing upon exposure, the sensitive individual experiences perhaps a headache, joint pain, muscle fatigue, or other symptoms several days later. The patient might have no idea that eating broccoli on Monday caused a headache or muscle pain by Thursday afternoon. This makes it more difficult to pinpoint the cause of the problem, and thus can lead to chronic and often unexplained diseases.

To my knowledge, the first writing about this immunologic phenomenon was by a nutritionist from Brooklyn, New York, named Peter D'Adamo. Many years ago, he published a book titled *Eat Right 4 Your Type*. It was a layperson's book written not for the scientific community but had relevance to anyone who was sick with a diagnosis not obvious to doctors.

Dr. D'Adamo writes that all people have in their blood small immune particles, which he calls "ligands," and these ligands are made by the immune system in response to exposure to a variety of foods. Some people have lots of such antibodies, and others have very few. He observed in his nutrition practice that rash, low-grade fever, muscle and joint pain, headaches, and a number of other symptoms in chronically ill people seemed to go away when they rotated off certain foods. The relief of symptoms often required a few weeks off the foods and certainly did not occur the first day the food was removed.

Over a period of time, Dr. D'Adamo recognized that people

with certain blood types had certain food sensitivities not present in those with other blood types. After years of working with patients, he—like his father before him—was sure that blood type influences the entire immune system, and that ligands directed against foods are important causes of various human diseases. He and his colleagues did not actually measure the ligands. They simply formulated a group of foods that people of a certain blood type should probably not eat and gave their patients a rotation schedule for the foods.

I'm sure this did not always work, but the idea was so intriguing that hundreds of thousands of people bought *Eat Right 4 Your Type* and put the process to use in their lives. Dr. D'Adamo's book organizes a number of foods into ten to twelve groups, designating several foods in each group that benefit persons of a certain blood type, and several foods that are potentially harmful and can cause symptoms in persons of that blood type.

About thirty years ago, one of my patients, an officer of a large company in San Antonio, gave me a copy of Dr. D'Adamo's book. He told me he was eating according to the plan and had lost about ten pounds, gotten rid of some bothersome headaches, and had seen a fifty-point drop in his serum cholesterol level—a goodly amount. He had eliminated from his diet only a handful of foods, and he couldn't believe what a change it had made in his life and overall health. I told him I would read the book and potentially tell other patients about it.

I asked several colleagues about the book and what they knew about IgG antibodies to food. Nobody had any knowledge of the topic. I more or less dismissed the idea as not very important clinically. My allergist friends affirmed that our blood has IgG antibodies directed against foods but that the antibodies do not actually cause any symptoms or diseases.

I was still intrigued by anything that could possibly make someone's serum cholesterol drop so significantly without medications. Several years later, I learned of a laboratory in Florida that measured IgG antibodies to about two hundred foods in a relatively simple and inexpensive assay. I thought to myself that these were the same ligands Dr. D'Adamo noted in *Eat Right 4 Your Type*. I ordered the test from Florida on my own blood because, if I remember correctly, the first test was free to me. The result came back that I was sensitive to several foods. I don't remember all of them, but cantaloupe and bananas, which I ate often and loved, were among the culprits. I stopped eating them for a couple of weeks and did not notice any change in how I felt. I should have checked my cholesterol and other lipids, but I did not.

A month or two later, however, I was seeing a patient who came to me with a chronic illness after having been to lots of doctors' offices but with little improvement of her symptoms. She was desperate, and I listened to her and deeply wanted to help her. She had been diagnosed with chronic fatigue and fibromyalgia, and had not gotten well despite changing her diet and taking a variety of prescription medications. With nothing else to do for her, I told her about the blood test from Florida. While I was doubtful it would help her, it seemed worth having her blood tested.

I must tell you she was very miserable. She had shut down her Mary Kay cosmetics business because of chronic muscle pain and terrible fatigue that kept her in bed many hours per day. She had no idea what was causing the problem. After praying with her, I gave instructions to have her blood drawn and sent to the lab in Florida.

When I received the results, I was embarrassed to have to share her results with her. My own test had revealed about ten positive foods to which I had an IgG antibody reaction. Her blood study revealed only one food: tomatoes. The reaction in the lab was quantified as very strong. Sheepishly, I called my patient with the result and apologized profusely that I was not able to help her much with the testing. To my surprise, when I told her about the tomato reaction at the lab, she told me tomatoes were her favorite food and that she ate them at least ten different ways almost every day. I told her it probably would not help, but I recommended she avoid tomatoes for a week or so to see what might happen. She admitted it would be difficult but agreed to try.

Amazingly, about a week later my patient told me her muscles no longer hurt, her chronic fatigue was gone, and several other bothersome symptoms had disappeared. I was amazed. How many other people were wandering around with a variety of symptoms related to the same mechanism but with no knowledge of it? I talked to a couple of my allergist friends, who assured me that IgG food antibody testing is of no clinical importance and that the result in my patient was likely psychosomatic. I wasn't convinced, however, because I had witnessed a relatively miraculous transformation in an ill woman who had little hope of getting well.

I realized at that moment something that had escaped me in medical school, residency, and nephrology fellowship. Allopathic medicine, which is what I practice and is taught in medical schools, deals with what happens when you apply a certain therapy or procedure on a good-sized group of people. If a specific result occurs, we always address whether or not the result is statistically significant. If it meets statistical significance, the procedure or medical treatment is said to work and is deemed valuable. If it does not meet statistical significance, it is determined that it does not work. That is how doctors are taught to think. It doesn't make any difference if a therapy seems to work on a selected individual patient. It is only considered to be of importance if it works on a statistically significant number in a group of people.

The problem with this way of thinking is that for my patient, something that doesn't work statistically in a large study group worked quite well for her as an individual. This realization during the 1980s led to my taking on a different view of the medicine I was practicing. It gave me freedom to try, with individual patients, varying approaches that did not appear to work in double-blind controlled medical studies—what we have come to expect from medical schools. I understand the reason and need for such academic thinking. It allows medical students to know what to do for sick people in general. It does not, however, show us how to be creative in treating one patient at a time.

During the past thirty years, several laboratories have been measuring IgG antibody reactions with sophisticated technology that can actually tell people whether they have positive antibody reactions against foods. The reports are colorful and informative, and the testing is not very expensive.

Allopathic medicine community members—many of whom are fine clinicians—continue to insist that dietary changes related to IgG antibody reactions to foods do not work in treating health issues. I suspect thousands of patients would beg to differ. At minimum, all should be aware of the controversy, and the knowledge that many individuals benefit from dietary approaches to personal health.

The complexity of blood types as connected to people's possible food allergies shows that the immune system functions in intricate and often unique ways. As the medical world ventured into organ transplants, it became abundantly clear

that blood type was not the immune system's only defense—
and if we wanted to understand and overcome the immune
system's rejection of transplanted organs, we would need to
make sacrifices.

CHAPTER THREE

THROUGH THE LENS OF TRANSPLANTS

The first kidney transplant was done from one identical twin to her sister. As might have been expected, the sister's kidney worked beautifully in the recipient because the sisters' immune systems were identical. The recipient's antibodies and white blood cells did not recognize her sister's kidney as foreign. As a result, the recipient did not need drugs or chemical manipulation of her immune system to allow her to receive a healthy, normally functioning kidney from her sister.

The next kidney transplant performed, however, did not fare as well. A non-identical twin set of sisters were the subjects. One had kidney failure and was on dialysis. Her twin sister agreed to donate a kidney, and the operation went well. For the first few days, the kidney worked fine, but then rather suddenly, the recipient's kidney function began to deteriorate. The patient was back on dialysis in less than two weeks. When the sister's kidney was removed, it was black and scarred-looking instead of the usual slightly purple and pink colors.

What had gone wrong? The recipient's immune system had after a day or two begun to recognize her non-identical sister's tissues as foreign, so antibodies and white blood cells were produced to attack the kidney—just like the immune system attacks germs.

If the donor and recipient of a kidney transplant were not identical twins but had compatible red cells matched for blood types A, B, AB, and O, and for Rh factor, one might assume all transplants would go very well. We clinicians who were there in the early days found out, of course, that blood typing was not enough to prevent organ rejection. Other previously unknown parts of the immune system stepped up, making it difficult to successfully transplant kidneys.

The key, therefore, was to suppress the immune system. The next time a non-related kidney transplant was attempted, doctors knew they had to give the recipient some kind of medication to poison the immune system and prevent rejection of the kidney. The only available chemical known to inhibit white blood cell and antibody activity was a steroid fairly similar in biochemistry to cortisol, which is made in the adrenal glands.

Cortisol was, by the 1950s, synthesized in laboratories and made available for doctors in tablet form or as an injectable medication. Cortisol in high dosage, given as a tablet called prednisone or methylprednisolone, had been shown in transplants on dogs and pigs to prevent rejection of transplanted kidneys—even in dogs and pigs of very different types. When the next kidney transplant of non-identical twins was undertaken, the recipient received a fairly high dose of the steroid medication (Medrol or prednisone).

Despite the two siblings being non-identical, the new kidney worked beautifully for weeks and weeks with stable kidney function and no rejection. Unfortunately, when the steroid dosage was reduced to prevent known side effects of the medication, the recipient's new kidney began to be destroyed—rejected—and kidney function diminished. When higher dosages of the steroid were given, the rejection process stopped and the kidney was saved.

OUR UNIQUE IMMUNOLOGY

One of the first breakthroughs in renal transplantation and that of other organs occurred when a new immunologic test was introduced in the early 1970s. It was called a crossmatch test, which was basically a laboratory analysis of whether a potential organ donor's white blood cells, or lymphocytes, could be destroyed by something in the serum of a potential recipient.

It turns out many of us have naturally occurring antibodies against the cells of other individuals. These are mostly IgG antibodies like those related to foods. In the early days of transplantation, physicians discovered they could measure whether a waiting recipient for a kidney transplant had preformed IgG antibodies against a potential donor. Serum from the potential recipient was obtained and placed in tiny wells in a laboratory dish. A known number of the potential donor's white blood cells were placed in the same wells. If the white cells became coagulated and destroyed in the next hour, the recipient was deemed to have a positive crossmatch against the potential donor. This meant the potential recipient had preformed antibodies against the potential donor.

Kidney transplant surgeons and nephrologists came to know early on that a positive crossmatch indicated a transplant would not work. The recipient would kill the donor kidney by rejection in a very short period of time, just as if the donor and recipient had different A, B, or O blood type discrepancies. This crossmatch knowledge became increasingly important as we began to see young kidney patients who had no family members as potential donors. The crossmatch test also helped us learn that many patients with kidney failure had preformed IgG antibodies against members of their families and therefore could not in many cases receive a kidney from a mother, father, or sibling.

We learned from the earliest days that people are immunologically very different from one another, even within families. Even among people who share blood types, DNA, and genetic relationships, immune systems vastly differ. Millions of variables—some of which we understand and some we are still discovering—interact to make us wholly unique. Understanding your health, both inside and outside of a clinical setting, requires you to appreciate this uniqueness. Template solutions may not always work for you. Flexibility, agility, and awareness are key. Just like with my patient whose chronic pain got better once she stopped eating tomatoes—whether it was psychosomatic or connected—it's impossible to know what will fall within the statistically significant section of the population and what won't.

The sheer range of this uniqueness became apparent with new testing called tissue typing. It was discovered that all of us have on our white blood cells (lymphocytes) small protein markers that make us unique and unlike other human beings. These protein markers, first identified in the 1960s, are known as HLA markers (Human Lymphocyte Antigens). Various proteins were identified and compartmentalized into two large groupings known as A and B. Even within the A and B groupings, many different protein structures were identified, but it was shown that each human being has only four of these structures—an A and a B marker from their mother, and an A and a B marker from their father.

In the 1970s, tissue typing was developed to test these HLA markers, and the results were astonishing. Since there are thirty to forty different A markers, and the same number of different B markers, there are a lot of possibilities for combinations in any individual. It is very unlikely that you and I, coming from two entirely different sets of parents, would have a matching set of four antigens on the surface of our lymphocytes.

Let's say your father's HLA tissue typing shows him to be HLA-A27, HLA-A34, HLA-B14, and HLA-B29. Your mother has an entirely different set of numbers—perhaps HLA-A6, HLA-A30, HLA-B23, and HLA-B41. When you were born, your father gave to you HLA-A27 and HLA-B14, while your mother gave you HLA-A6 and HLA-B23. Your tissue typing would show you to be A6, A27, B23, and B14. You have these HLA markers throughout your life, and they influence the success of a prospective transplant of kidney, lung, liver, heart, or other organs from you to another person or vice versa.

How important is this typing? I was astounded when I first reviewed the numbers. Let's say you have a sibling whose typing is A34, A30, B29, and B41. You and your sibling, who came from the same set of parents, have no HLA antigens in common. This is called a zero antigen match—or a total mismatch. Siblings can receive the same HLA antigens from each parent, no antigens in common (like the above example), or two antigens in common—for instance, the same two from one parent but a different two from the other.

When we began doing transplants from unrelated parties—usually referred to then as cadaver transplants because the kidneys came from those who were killed in auto accidents—we found that HLA typing was critically important in determining whether or not the recipient would likely reject the donated kidney. Because kidney rejection is such a severe process that ultimately leads to loss of a donated kidney—and occasionally to loss of life—HLA typing to determine donor and recipient likeness became important as we attempted to do cadaver transplants, which are now called non-related kidney transplants.

We found that an HLA identical transplant (four antigen match) from one sibling to another yields a nearly 100 percent five-year survival of transplanted kidneys. What was called a one haplotype match—two antigens matched and the other two were mismatched—yielded a five-year transplant success rate of about 80 percent. In a half-matched HLA relationship between two siblings, about 20 percent of transplanted kidneys would be dead from rejection in less than five years. That is a pretty good success rate for someone on dialysis and in need of a kidney, but it certainly is not as good as the expected result from an HLA identical sibling-to-sibling match.[4]

How about a parent-to-child or child-to-parent kidney donation? Since a child can receive only one pair of HLA antigens from each parent, the best a child could expect from a parental transplanted organ would be a two-antigen match. The only exception to this would be if both parents share one or more A or B antigens. If this were to occur—which it does occasionally—there could be a three-antigen match in a parent-to-child or child-to-parent transplant.

As more parent-to-child or child-to-parent transplants were accomplished, we learned that the expected success rate was about 80/20. Eighty percent of donated kidneys would still be

---

4   This information ultimately led to a national data bank that contains tissue typing data for all dialysis patients who have been approved for transplantation but have no donor. With this information widely available, a kidney dialysis patient from New York can receive a perfectly matched kidney from a deceased donor in Los Angeles if the logistics and transportation can be worked out. Widespread tissue typing has therefore been a great blessing to many who would not otherwise have been able to obtain a transplant in their local area.

working in five years, and 20 percent would be rejected and dead. I might add here that rejection of a transplanted kidney does not equal death of the patient who rejected the kidney. Because of the success of dialysis, patients who reject kidneys simply return to dialysis and await the opportunity to receive another kidney transplant in the future.

What about totally HLA mismatched kidneys—four antigen mismatched siblings or so-called cadaver kidneys? The success rate of this type of matching yielded a success rate of about 60/40. Sixty percent of such kidneys would still be working five years post-transplant, and the other 40 percent would be rejected. We learned also that the amount of antirejection medication needed to prevent rejection in totally mismatched kidneys was considerably greater than that needed in a better matched sibling-to-sibling, parent-to-child, or child-to-parent kidney transplant.

We also learned over the years that there were other protein markers on our white blood cells besides the A, B, O system and the HLA system, but these two systems continue to be the most important. The next most important antigen locus is called the D Locus, and it is important for typing but not as important as the systems mentioned above. Yet it is another protein marker on the white blood cells that can stimulate immune activity and cause rejection of transplanted organs.

I want people to appreciate the complexity of the human immune system and how delicately it differs among individuals. I also want us to appreciate the role the immune system plays in health. While our early experiences with transplantation taught that we could use drugs of various kinds to overcome the strength of the immune system—both the antibody system and the cellular system—we also learned there was a price to pay for the immunosuppression these agents cause.

THE PRICE PAID

Cortisol as an immunosuppressant helped the first non-twin organ transplant become successful. Our bodies make these same steroid chemicals each day, and they are necessary for life. The problem is that the amount of steroid of that type that we make in our adrenal glands each day is pretty minimal. The amount needed to prevent rejection of a transplanted kidney is at least two to three times what a healthy human being is expected to produce daily. Unfortunately, at the dosage needed to prevent rejection, the steroids cause some unacceptable side effects.

We had known for a number of years prior to the first kidney transplants that high doses of corticosteroids—mostly prednisone or Medrol—are harmful. Back before the 1940s, some patients were found to have tumors of the adrenal gland cortex. These tumors produced very large amounts of cortisol. These patients were pretty easy to diagnose if the tumor had been present for a long time and the disease was well developed.

The excess production of cortisol creates a condition called Cushing's Disease, which is named after the physician who first described the condition. A typical patient with Cushing's Disease presents with high blood pressure, obesity, increased hairiness, diabetes, a very puffy face, acne, osteoporosis, severe muscular weakness (especially in the quadriceps muscles), thinned-out skin with bruising, cataracts in the eyes, and various infections. Interestingly, if the tumor of the adrenal gland is surgically removed, the entire clinical syndrome, with all of its complications and side effects, disappears over time. As more and more patients with Cushing's Disease were treated successfully with surgical removal of the tumor, it became apparent that overproduction of cortisol and other steroid hormones from the adrenal glands is a dangerous clinical situation.

The most ominous of side effects from overproduction of cortisol is the increase in infections. Patients with Cushing's Disease have an increase not only in normal infections like skin infections, pneumonia, and sinus infections, but also unusual infections such as fungal diseases, parasitic diseases, and some viral diseases as well as a number of malignancies. Cushing's Disease showed us that increased production of cortisol and other adrenal steroids leads to a decrease in immune function, which makes patients vulnerable to infections and malignancies.

When laboratories in the 1950s were able to produce cortisol and make it available as a tablet or injectable medicine, doctors were wary of the medicine's potency and potential dangers. But they knew successful transplantation was possible only when they suppressed the immune system, and cortisol was the only available drug to do so at the time. Only with nearly toxic doses of cortisol could the recipient of a transplant hope to prevent rejection of the organ. Early recipients of kidney transplants were forced to accept many dangerous side effects of excess corticosteroids for the privilege of having a working kidney.

During those early years of high-dose steroid use, almost all of our transplanted patients, after receiving a new kidney from a sibling, experienced unbelievable weight gain and developed Type 2 diabetes, worsening elevations of blood pressure, and osteoporosis of the spine and hips. The latter led to many patients requiring hip replacements, even in those as young as twenty years of age. By the time I was working with kidney transplant patients in the early 1970s, everyone knew we had to develop pharmacologic agents other than corticosteroids to prevent rejection of transplanted organs.

Thankfully, by the mid-1970s, God gave us a new drug, azathioprine (Imuran), which when used along with steroids allowed far lower doses of prednisone to prevent the rejection of transplanted kidneys. Imuran was a once-per-day pill that was easy for patients to swallow and caused few, if any, acute side effects.

It was soon discovered that the addition of Imuran to steroids in preventing rejection—even in HLA well-matched donors—led to a large increase in malignancies in kidney recipients. We sadly learned that risk of lymphomas and all kinds of solid organ tumors was fifty to one hundred times greater in kidney transplant patients who were receiving combination antirejection therapy. To me, this was unacceptable. It would be better, I thought, for the patient to remain on dialysis than to have a working kidney and then die of a rare cancer.

After Imuran came cyclosporine, which had the unique side effect of causing kidney damage, and its blood levels had to be carefully monitored to prevent the drug from injuring transplanted kidneys. A decade later another once-a-day drug, this one called PROGRAF, followed. Finally, an agent known as CellCept emerged from research laboratories a couple of decades ago, and it was found to work about the same on the immune system as did Imuran but with less long-term toxicity.

All these drugs decrease the capacity of the immune system to kill certain unusual germs. Skin infections with staph aureus had to be treated aggressively to prevent systemic severe infections. Patients with working kidney transplants often developed unusual infections with fungi like Cryptococcus, Histoplasma, or Candida. How sad it was to see a young patient with a working kidney transplant die of cryptococcal meningitis. We had to be especially vigilant in looking for cancer and weird infections, as well as common infections, in patients taking immunosuppressive medications.

THE VALUE OF THE IMMUNE SYSTEM

One of the most powerful stories of just how important the immune system is in protecting us comes from the 1970s, when I was a nephrologist in the US Air Force. A well-known kidney transplant program at that time was treating a twenty-year-old man who had kidney failure secondary to immune damage to his kidneys. He was on dialysis and had no siblings. Because his mother had high blood pressure, she was not an acceptable donor. His father was a healthy man but had developed prostate cancer a few years earlier and after prostate surgery was not deemed to be a good donor either.

The patient therefore waited a couple of years for a non-related kidney transplant, but his number never came up and no transplant was done. After a few years, the issue came up again as to whether his father might be a good kidney donor after all. The father was reevaluated, and he was healthy with no signs of cancer. The transplant was done successfully, and the young man was out of the dialysis clinic and free to travel for the first time in years. He remained healthy for a few months but soon developed a cough. He was treated with several antibiotics, but they did not have a positive effect on his cough. His kidney function was perfect.

A chest X-ray done after a few weeks revealed several large nodules in his lungs bilaterally. His physicians wondered if it was a fungal infection but decided to proceed with a biopsy of the nodules. The biopsy revealed prostate cancer. He had inadvertently received a transplanted focus of prostate cancer from his father along with the kidney transplant.

The father's immune system, which was healthy, was able to easily fight off the cancer and keep him in remission. But the son's immune system, which was damaged by the immunosuppressants we were giving him to ensure the kidney transplant worked, couldn't function well enough to keep the cancer at bay so the disease got a foothold in his body. What a dilemma!

The patient needed a working immune system to keep the cancer from spreading, but stopping the immunosuppressant medication would also definitely lead to rejection of the new kidney. After a short time, his physicians felt the patient's only hope was to stop his antirejection medicines—Imuran and steroids. This would lead to rejection of the prostate cancer in his lungs, and in fact, that is exactly what happened. The patient rejected his father's kidney but also rejected his father's prostate cancer. His lungs cleared, and his cough went away.

I tell you this lest you think suppressing the immune system is the best way forward for all treatments. The immune system takes care of us to a degree we often do not appreciate, and damaging or suppressing it can lead to severe consequences. This was a tremendous learning experience for all the physicians involved with this patient and his father, as the relationship between the human immune system and cancer was so evident. The human body is more intricate and unique than we can fully grasp, despite our many medical leaps.

Now that you have a better understanding of the human immune system's complexity and our immunological uniqueness, let's look at how precisely the immune system interacts with germs. Understanding this process of interaction unlocks many surprising discoveries about the root causes of illness—and the biome that live in the tube.

PART TWO

CHAPTER FOUR

THE IMMUNE SYSTEM AND GERMS

The first part of this book explores how the immune system was created to save us from various microorganisms, to prevent the introduction of foreign tissues into the blood—like mismatched red blood cells and kidney transplants—and to prevent foreign environmental chemicals from entering the body. This understanding, while it may seem simple, is the foundation behind many diseases of unknown causes, and this chapter details how so.

Over the course of my career, I realized that many diseases are created by the immune system's interaction with bacteria or yeast in the bowels—what the immune system perceives as invaders or germs, including diseases in the lungs, kidneys, hearts, and much more. I'll unpack this statement gradually in the chapters that follow, taking you on a journey of how I made these discoveries—and how I had to break away from traditional medical thinking to do so.

Let's begin with the foundational premise on which this

argument is based and that has been proven through clinical experiments: the immune system's reaction to germs can cause disease in distant organs that are far from the site of infection.

KIDNEY IMMUNE DISEASE: HUNTING FOR CAUSES

I performed biopsies on kidneys for the first time when I was a nephrology fellow in the US Air Force. I learned that various diseases can injure kidneys and that, for the most part, we didn't have the slightest idea what caused these problems.

We *did* know through biopsy that many diseases that caused loss of kidney function appeared to be related to an inflammatory process in the kidney—not dissimilar from the inflammation that occurs when one has a sore throat, skin infection, or other minor ailment. These other kinds of kidney disease seemed to be connected to the immune system. All were called glomerulonephritis, because the kidney's basic filter plant, glomerulus, had "itis," or inflammation.

Treatment for these immune-mediated kidney diseases basically involved steroids or other immunosuppressive medicines administered to patients who had diseases thought to be caused by the immune system. All of these drugs in some way or another killed off the immune system—just like we learned to do to prevent rejection of transplanted kidneys and hearts. The television commercials I discuss at the beginning of this book are a testament to the same phenomenon.

What bothered me over the years was that no one ever seemed to have the faintest idea why the "itis" was occurring in the glomerulus. We knew only that the poor kidney was inflamed and figured it was bad luck that it happened. Most of the time, all we could do to treat it was—you guessed it—give corticosteroids to try to shut off the inflammation.

But we know the cause for *one* immune kidney disease—and that cause may be the clue to why other named immune-mediated kidney diseases occur. Let's look at a strange experiment with a rabbit and a strep infection.

RABBIT AND THE STREP INFECTION

Nearly seventy-five years ago, as bacteriology became a better science, and we began to recognize various common bacteria and how they act, a group of pioneering nephrologists studied what became known as post-streptococcal glomerulonephritis. It was well known that children who had a streptococcus infection in their throats often later developed symptoms in other organs, including the heart valves and kidneys. Even after there was no more strep infection in the throat or other locations, kidney function often deteriorated to the point that the child was in kidney failure. Prior to dialysis in the late 1950s, this disease meant certain death for the patient.

Physicians conducted studies in which they inoculated strep bacteria into the skin and soft tissues of the leg of a rabbit. The animal's body had the expected inflammatory response in the infected tissue, and a small abscess developed. About ten days later, with no spread of the infection, the investigators found protein and blood in the rabbit's urine. Blood tests to measure kidney function showed loss of cleaning of the blood, and the process led to total kidney failure within a couple of weeks. Upon autopsy of the rabbit, no evidence of strep infection was found in the kidney. The strep was only in the skin of the leg of the animal.

The investigators concluded that the kidney damage occurred because of something in the blood being connected to the strep infection in the animal's skin. Over time, after many more rabbit autopsies, it was concluded that the rabbits' immune systems were making some kind of chemicals in response to the strep bacteria, and that those immune chemicals were cross-reacting with the kidney and destroying the kidney as well as the strep in the abscesses on the rabbits' legs.

It turned out the strep bacteria had some unique structural characteristics that made it similar enough to the structure of a human kidney that an immune reaction against the strep caused an immune reaction in a distant site far from the streptococcal infection. I wondered why this did not happen with other types of bacterial infections leading to damage in distant places, in other organs. No one talked about this idea, so I put the thoughts away—at least for a time.

Streptococcus, a fairly common skin bacteria that also gets into the throat and upper airways, can induce the immune system to attack other parts of the body as well—including joint cartilage and heart valves. Prior to having penicillin and other antibiotics to kill the streptococcus, thousands of people with strep throat or other strep infections developed rheumatic fever. This disease, which is rarely seen anymore, was characterized by fever, rash, joint pain, and heart murmurs caused by damaged cardiac valves. The mitral valve, between the left atrium and left ventricle, was one of the main damage sites. The strep bacteria did not infect the valves or joints. The streptococcus instead seemed to set in motion an immunologic cascade that created chemical damage to the heart valves, skin, and joints.

After the development of penicillin and other antibacterial medicines in the 1940s, rheumatic fever decreased in importance and slowly disappeared from physicians' offices. I suspect that it is a rare cardiologist or primary care physician who has seen even one case of rheumatic fever today. Why? Because when people show up at the doctor's office with a sore throat, the physician or nurse typically does a throat culture or strep test. The latter takes only a few minutes and tells the clinician if any streptococcus bacteria are growing in the throat. If the test is positive for strep, the physician typically prescribes penicillin, a cephalosporin, or some other antibiotic to kill the strep.

HEART VALVES AND KIDNEY DISEASE

The experiment with the rabbit and strep infection proves that immune reactions to germs can cause disease in distant organs that are far from the site of the infection. Another example proves the same hypothesis—and demonstrates how the healthcare industry, structured as it is, can miss the underlying cause.

During my years as a hospital-based nephrologist, I had opportunity from time to time to care for patients who had developed infections of one or more heart valves. This unusual illness is called subacute bacterial endocarditis. It is subacute because its symptoms develop over a number of weeks or even months, and it often causes no symptoms at all for quite a long time in those who develop the illness. Although streptococcus bacteria can cause such an infection, it usually does not—at least not during most of the past forty years.

Most current cardiac valve infections occur when skin bacteria from an intravenous line or skin surgical site enter into the bloodstream and spread through veins to the heart. Although this sort of infection probably happens quite frequently, only rarely do the bacteria get stuck on the surface of the heart valve and damage the valve. The infection part of the equation occurs most often when something is already wrong with the valve. The patient may have a heart murmur that was detected over the years but was deemed not to cause any pumping problems for the heart.

When bacteria, fungi, and other organisms get into the blood and attach to the abnormal valve surface, a valve infection can develop. Over time, the valve might fail, causing congestive heart failure and other cardiac complications. It often takes an infection a number of months to create much damage to the valve, but eventually injury occurs and cardiac symptoms develop.

The germ that currently causes such infections is usually a staphylococcus, unusual strep organism, or sometimes even a fungus or germ from the colon or small bowel. The patient may come to the doctor with night sweats, low-grade fever, and malaise. Almost any doctor would suspect possible infection. I saw a number of patients, however, who presented to their doctors with joint pain, rash, and evidence of inflammation of their kidneys—not very different from the patients who had rheumatic fever due to strep infection.

A patient who presented with bilateral joint pain was thought to possibly have rheumatoid arthritis or another rheumatologic disease. If a patient presented with numbness in his feet or a rash, the primary care physician usually made a referral to a dermatologist or neurologist for further evaluation. With protein and blood in urine, the patient typically ended up in the office of a nephrologist like me. In such a circumstance, I thought the patient had some kind of immune kidney disease with damage occurring at the level of the filtration areas of the kidneys—glomerulonephritis. If I listened to the patient's heart and heard a loud murmur, my mind turned to thinking about the patient's heart as the source of the kidney disease.

Over the years of my practice, I saw eight to ten such patients. In each case an accurate diagnosis was not made until the patient had been sick for quite a long time. The true cause of the patient's blood and protein in the urine was indeed nephritis, but the kidney inflammation was caused by an infection on a heart valve, not an infection in the kidneys.

How did this happen? There was no infection in the kidney in any of these cases. The infection was on a cardiac valve. Just as in the case of post-streptococcal kidney disease, the patient's immune system was responding to the valve infection, and other tissues—skin, joints, nerves, kidney—were secondarily injured.

Eventually the correct diagnosis would be made by a cardiologist who performed an echocardiogram and identified the infectious process—usually called a "vegetation" (little growth) on the cardiac valve. Even then, the cardiologist would not know which germ was causing the infection until the laboratory identified the organism on a culture of the patient's blood drawn during a bout of fever and chills.

Just like with the rabbit and the strep infection, other infections on other types of organisms can result in triggering of the immune system and development of symptoms in organs that are not infected. This is the fundamental principle for the chapters that follow.

NEXT STEPS

I have come to believe that almost all chronic disease has a background related to immune system activity, like that described previously. Most disease is not caused by the streptococcus, although that was the model studied so many years ago and is still widely accepted by academic physicians. The truth is that many different microorganisms, such as yeast and bacteria, can cause immunologic disease.

I believe microflora do not affect all people equally, due to our immunological uniqueness, which influences how the immune system interacts with these germs. Differences in genetics—even those discussed in the section on tissue typing—can determine who develops adult asthma, fibromyalgia, chronic fatigue, rheumatoid arthritis, glomerulonephritis, and a host of other diseases with strange names and no known causes.

Something causes these diseases. Getting it right requires new ways of thinking and courage in those who are bold enough to think differently. Even though I had been practicing medicine for ten years, I had a lot of learning left to do in the 1980s, and I might never have realized it had a patient not gifted me a book.

CHAPTER FIVE

THE YEAST WITHIN US

My understanding of diseases caused by the immune system took a huge leap during the early 1980s. I was working late most nights, taking care of patients with horrible illnesses. I was growing tired of often hopeless problems and lots of death. Unexpectedly, a patient gave me a copy of a book titled *The Yeast Connection*. I confessed I had not heard of it, but to be polite, I told him I would look at it. The patient pulled a copy of the book out of his briefcase and handed it to me. If he had not done so, I'm sure I would never have looked for the book or considered reading it. I'm very thankful I did, however, because that book and several others like it changed the fundamental way in which I viewed patients and their diseases.

Before I share about *The Yeast Connection*, I must first explain why as a young physician I would not have read this book or others like it. My explanation shines a light on a way of thinking that dominates much of the medical profession today. That needs to change if we are to step away from expensive and harmful treatments that don't fix the underlying cause of disease.

THE FORMATION OF MEDICAL THOUGHT

After medical school, we doctors read only material that comes from medical research done only in reputable medical schools and hospitals all over the world. We learn to recognize good and bad research, and are proud to know the difference. The average kid who comes to medical school does not know a lot about medicine, disease, medications, or the causes of diseases and how to treat them. There is an incredible amount to learn, and no medical student is expected to read anything except what comes from a reputable institution.

I personally have relied on the *New England Journal of Medicine* as my major source of information, having subscribed to this famous journal since 1967. Published for nearly two hundred years, *NEJM* has been a major source of believable information for that entire time. There are many other medical publications, of course, but *NEJM* has been my teacher.

The point is that young physicians get information from those who have gone before them and primarily from academic institutions that publish articles in reputable journals like *NEJM*. A talented editorial board reviews what is published in all such journals, determining which articles practicing physicians get to read. Many physicians who do basic research related to human disease do not necessarily see sick people but spend much time reading what others write and setting up studies to see what happens when a patient with such-and-such disease takes such-and-such medication for such-and-such a time.

Studies are set up and published by those who often have not taken care of sick people for extended periods of time and whose jobs are dependent upon their turning out new papers that lead to personal fame, and fame for the department, hospital, or medical school where they work.

In my early years of medicine, I took care of the people

in whatever hospital I was stationed, read a little about their diseases, and talked to those who had gone before me and seen more cases than I had. I was excited just to know the names of diseases and to tell the patient the name of the disease I was diagnosing. I didn't think much about the causes, because I was so proud just to identify the disease. This, unfortunately, happens to many physicians.

The problem has been compounded during the past fifty years with medical and surgical sub-specialization. In the mid-1970s, when I entered hospital-based medicine as a budding nephrologist, a family practice doctor usually came by to see hospitalized patients each day. The family practice doctor got in the habit of occasionally asking a subspecialist like me to see his patient and offer advice about how to fix whatever was broken. The best and smartest doctors at that time, in my opinion, were cardiologists. They knew everything about hearts and were very good internal medicine doctors as well, knowing a good deal about everything an internal medicine doctor is supposed to know.

Gradually over the next couple of decades, cardiologists generally became doctors who did surgical procedures, such as putting little wires into people's hearts to make them better, for the express purpose of making a living. Unfortunately, many cardiologists became less astute at the other aspects of internal medicine. The deep-thinking cardiologists of the 1960s and 1970s slowly disappeared. Taking care of the whole patient became someone else's domain.

Unfortunately, the family practice doctors of those early days were on their way out as well. These primary care family physicians accepted the apparent desire of educated patients to have a subspecialist for almost any kind of medical problem. Even general internal medicine doctors bought in to the game, expecting a urologist to do the urology, a nephrologist to do the nephrology, a cardiologist to do the cardiology, and an ENT doctor to fix anything broken in the sinuses. After a time, there were few doctors who took care of the whole person or thought deeply about fundamental causes of disease. The medical community simply accepted the dogma that such-and-such disease is of unknown cause, it is treated with such-and-such medicine, and with this treatment it has a such-and-such percent chance of getting well.

The result, forty years later, is a primary care system that is badly broken. Essentially, the old general practice doctor who dominated the scene in the 1960s is gone away, and the care of patients is relegated to a team of medical and surgical subspecialists. Many of these specialists do not know or understand very well what other medical and surgical subspecialists know and believe. Common knowledge sometimes does not cross over from one specialty to another. This sad dynamic is responsible for many of medicine's exorbitant costs and the general public's dissatisfaction with individual medical care. I was there in the 1970s, proud to be able to identify some diseases and make a diagnosis, but I was not very good at understanding what went wrong to cause the disease.

The Yeast Connection changed the equation for me.

THE YEAST CONNECTION

The Yeast Connection: A Medical Breakthrough was written by a physician named William G. Crook, who had never been published in the *New England Journal of Medicine*. What he wrote about probably would never be published in *NEJM* or any other good journal, because his ideas on how to make some patients get well would likely not work in a high enough percentage of patients to achieve statistical significance. If it doesn't have statistical significance, it doesn't work at all. That, of course, is a lie, but prior to reading *The Yeast Connection*, I didn't know it was a lie. *The Yeast Connection* opened a new way of thinking for me in this regard.

What did Dr. Crook write in his book that got my attention and changed my thinking?

As I understand it, William G. Crook was a family practice doctor in Alabama. He was taking care of run-of-the-mill concerns doctors see in their offices. One common medical problem back in the '60s—and still somewhat of a problem—was female patients experiencing vaginal yeast infections. Doctors had recognized, almost since the development of penicillin in the late 1930s, that people who took antibiotics often developed thrush in their mouths, diarrhea, or for many women, vaginal yeast infections.

Yeast growing in the mouth creates a white mucous material that lines the cheeks and is irritating to the gingiva and other mucous membranes in the mouth. It is called thrush, and left untreated, it can lead to inflammation of the esophagus, cheeks, or tongue and to bleeding from this tube or the other inflamed areas. We learned to treat the problem in the mouth with a liquid preparation containing a topical agent called nystatin. Patients were instructed to swish, gargle, and swallow to coat the inner lining of the mouth with the medicine. Most of the time, after twelve to twenty-four hours of swishing and swallowing, the yeast growing in the mouth was dead, and the symptoms in the mouth went away. Patients continued taking the liquid medicine for about a week, and symptoms usually did not return—especially if the patient had finished the course of penicillin, which brought on the thrush.

In the early days of prescribing penicillin, many doctors also gave their patients a prescription for nystatin to hopefully prevent thrush. Sometime in the 1960s, someone wrote a scientific paper suggesting it was no longer necessary to give nystatin concomitantly with penicillin, since it didn't change outcomes sufficiently to merit the expense of giving the nystatin. Based on this single study, doctors stopped prescribing the two medicines together.

This is a classic case of what often happens with doctors. If someone writes a paper stating a treatment is no longer necessary, large groups of doctors tell one another it is not necessary, and a change in medical behavior occurs. In the case of yeast overgrowth leading to oral thrush or vaginal infections, many physicians essentially forgot that antibiotic use could be the cause of the problem. New prescriptions for new antibiotics were written, but concomitant use of nystatin ceased to be a common treatment.

In the 1960s, a number of other very potent antibiotics were developed that likely led to a worsening of the abovementioned biologic problem. Ampicillin, Amoxicillin, cephalosporins, fluoroquinolones, macrolides, and other bacteria-killing drugs came to be commonly used, but doctors did not typically elect to give nystatin to their patients, due to the scientific paper deeming it unnecessary. The academic assumption was that treating the potential increase in yeast growth wasn't very important, and that if it were, everyone would be doing it. Some patients who took these antibiotics developed thrush in their mouths, and some women developed vaginal thrush, or vaginal yeast infections. When this happened, most doctors prescribed an antifungal agent like nystatin, but only until symptoms of the yeast infection had dissipated.

In the 1960s, pharmaceutical companies, recognizing the importance of this problem for women who took strong antibiotics, developed suppositories that could be placed on an applicator and inserted into the vagina to treat vaginal yeast infections. Physicians and those in the pharmaceutical industry knew nystatin was unique in that it was not absorbed through mucous membranes into the bloodstream but effective only externally in treating surface infections in the mouth or vagina.

Nystatin is a nonabsorbable antifungal antibiotic that slides from the mouth down into the intestine and finally all the way to the anal canal without getting into the blood. Any nystatin in the mouth or vagina, therefore, remains in place and accomplishes its antifungal activity locally on the surface where it is placed, thus limiting its side effects. This made it a very good treatment for thrush in the mouth or vagina. Dr. Crook, with considerable wisdom and attention to detail, used this nonabsorbability of nystatin to make some rather startling observations.

Dr. Crook, like most family physicians, gave prescribed lots of nystatin suppositories to women who were taking Amoxicillin or Ampicillin. The suppositories were effective, but the treatment was messy and cumbersome, as most women weren't very enamored with the thought of putting the suppository in place. Dr. Crook, knowing nystatin could be taken by mouth, and that it was totally nonabsorbable and didn't cause side effects when taken orally, put some of his patients on oral nystatin in liquid or tablet form. When he did this, he decided to continue the anti-yeast therapy for several months to see if it prevented development of vaginal yeast overgrowth over the long term.

Much to his pleasure, and certainly that of his patients, the incidence of yeast infections during antibiotic use was remarkably reduced over the months that followed. This made him think the nystatin had somehow decreased the total volume of yeast organisms (mostly candida species) and that with low total volume of yeast in the bowel, there must be low total volume of yeast organisms in the vagina as well. This effect seemed to continue for many months, even after oral nystatin was discontinued. Eventually, the problem with yeast infection in the mouth or vagina would return, but often after a time lag of many months or even a couple of years.

This by itself would have been enough for him to recommend that all his patients who were taking antibiotics should consider a course of nystatin at the same time. But Dr. Crook made even more startling discoveries about the effects of nystatin taken orally.

In his book, Dr. Crook describes a patient who had been taking nystatin for some time and was elated that she had not experienced any further vaginal yeast infections. She added that an eczema rash on her hands and arms also had gone away while she was taking the nystatin. This got Dr. Crook's attention. Dr. Crook assured his patient that nystatin could not possibly have anything to do with her eczema rash going away, because nystatin does not get into the skin and therefore could not treat eczema. The patient insisted the rash had been present for several years and that it seemed to go away within a couple of weeks of her taking the nystatin.

Dr. Crook, while he poo-pooed the possible relationship, didn't forget what the patient had said. A few weeks later, another patient came back for a visit and reported that she, too, had not had a vaginal yeast infection for some time. She also mentioned that a chronic cough she had experienced for a number of months disappeared shortly after she began taking the nystatin tablets. Dr. Crook was quick to let her know this medicine could not possibly be responsible for making her cough go away, because nystatin does not get absorbed into the body and go to the lungs. She replied that she didn't care how it worked, but that she was very grateful to not be coughing. Dr. Crook didn't think much about the common thread between these two patients, but he fortunately did not totally forget.

Sometime later, another patient told him her headaches had gone away while she was taking "this nystatin stuff that you gave me."

By this time, Dr. Crook asked himself, "How can this be?" How could a medicine that does not enter the bloodstream from the gut possibly do anything to influence one patient getting well from a cough, another from a rash, and yet another from a headache?

He didn't understand it, but as the months went by and more patients came into his office with miraculous cures of all sorts of illnesses—all while they were taking nystatin to prevent vaginal yeast infections—Dr. Crook began to think outside the box. He hypothesized that somehow the yeast that grows routinely in all bowels can influence health in various parts of the body, and that the process can cause symptoms in a variety of locations. This didn't make much sense, because there was obviously no yeast in the head, skin, joints, or lungs. No—the yeast was only in the bowel, and somehow the yeast in the bowel was influencing symptoms in other locations.

But how? Dr. Crook wisely hypothesized that the yeast organisms routinely growing inside the bowel can sometimes, in some people, cause pathology in places far from the gut. He assumed that the host's immune system must have something to do with what he was observing. He did not know how it worked, but his assumption was that some change in the bowel occurred to induce formerly nontoxic yeast organisms to trigger the immune system to make chemicals that caused symptoms in various locations. When his patients took nystatin prophylactically to prevent vaginal yeast infections, it apparently reduced the amount of yeast also growing in the bowel and thus cleared up *all* symptoms the yeast was causing, including those occurring through its unexpected effect on the immune system in the bowel.

Dr. Crook again hypothesized that for the yeast to affect the immune system and create numerous symptoms in a given individual, there had to be some change either in the number of yeast organisms per square inch of bowel, or some fundamental change in the bowel to allow the normal amount of yeast per square inch to become toxic to the host. Otherwise, there should be no reason for the new symptom—whether a cough, headache, or rash.

Dr. Crook tried various dietary interventions to see if they would influence improvement in patients' symptoms. He already suspected that yeast grows more luxuriously in food principally composed of carbohydrates—yeast has to be added to grape juice to give us wine. His experiments in this regard were not always positive, but he felt certain that diet in some way influenced what was growing in the large and small intestines of his patients—diet had at least some influence on the number or activity of bowel yeast.

This was long before anyone in academic medicine knew the words *biome* or *probiotic*. I never once heard either of these words in medical school. I didn't know that about one thousand different species of microorganisms reside in the tube, and that each is unique and has its own life story. All species of microorganisms manufacture chemicals that protect them from one another. I never heard any of this in medical school nor during an excellent residency program in internal medicine. I guess that is why Dr. Crook found his findings to be so fascinating—he presumably hadn't heard of these concepts either.

Ultimately, he wrote down stories of many of his patients and how they seemed to get well from a variety of diseases when he treated them with a low-carb diet and nystatin. He sometimes treated patients with the strong antifungal agent fluconazole, but he usually stuck with nystatin because it seemed to work in a variety of situations without many side effects. He published his work in his book, *The Yeast Connection*, in 1968. It was one of those layperson's health books people read when sitting in an airport or the barber shop.

STATISTICAL SIGNIFICANCE

I'm sure many thoughtful people read the book and wondered if Dr. Crook's observations had any real importance. As a busy physician, I did not have time to read such stuff. Remember that we doctors choose to learn only from what is published in revered medical journals—and even then, only when it is interesting to us and relevant to our daily practices. I'm sure double-blind controlled studies of nystatin versus yeast were performed sometime after Dr. Crook's book was published. Such studies undoubtedly showed that if anyone got better with nystatin and a low-carbohydrate diet that it was by chance alone and not really related to the nystatin or the diet. In short, it didn't have statistical significance.

If I had read the book as a medical student, I would have told you nystatin does not work. According to standards set by statistically relevant medical science, I would have been correct. If I had read a paper that claimed treatment of a cough, rash, joint pain, or headache might include nystatin, I would have said there was strong evidence that it did not work and would not ever have written the prescription. In essence, therapies may be very helpful to individuals but never get put into widespread practice because doctors are told these treatments don't work according to good statistical criteria. This is exactly what happened when Dr. Crook wrote *The Yeast Connection*. People read it and maybe gave it to their doctors, who likely did not read it, and the concept was soon forgotten.

Luckily, though, I read *The Yeast Connection*, and it changed my medical practice.

CHAPTER SIX

YEAST AND DISEASES

By the early 1980s, I was taking care of hundreds of people with kidney failure. Some were in my dialysis clinics, receiving three-times-per-week dialysis to clean their blood of metabolic impurities. Others were in hospitals, receiving dialysis and other therapies for the entire range of human disease. Most of my patients in South Texas had diabetes, having suffered various ravages of this disease for many years. They developed all complications of diabetes while in my care. This included almost any pathologic condition that can possibly occur in almost any organ.

My various patients, in addition to having kidney failure caused by diabetes, also had blindness, all kinds of cardiac disease, atherosclerotic plaque disease of arteries in every known organ system, liver disease, lung disease, malignancies of all kinds, and amputations of fingers, toes, legs, and arms. The healthiest patients underwent kidney transplants, and I was blessed to care for many of them as well. This isn't to say I am such a great doctor. It is only to let you know I was blessed to see almost everything that can medically occur in the daily life of patients with kidney, heart, lung, or liver disease, and to be involved in the daily care of such patients.

Thanks to one patient, I picked up Dr. Crook's book and read it. I read of the miraculous improvement in symptoms of many diseases. I knew that many of my sick patients on dialysis had unexplained symptoms, and I wondered if Dr. Crook's process of prescribing nystatin might help some of my patients. I said to myself, "Every day I give my patients medicines that are expensive and toxic and cause a variety of side effects. Here is a guy telling me that maybe my patient's rash or headaches or joint pain or cough might be treatable with a nonabsorbable, nontoxic medicine that costs ten dollars per month."

I decided to give it a try with patients who had chronic symptoms that were unresponsive to whatever medicine I had prescribed to provide relief thus far.

MY FIRST TRY WITH NYSTATIN

I had three middle-aged women dialysis patients in the Uvalde, Texas, dialysis clinic—all of whom had a dry nonproductive cough for at least three months. The cough was of unknown cause and had not responded to at least two courses of antibiotics and a variety of prescription and over-the-counter medicines that typically suppress persistent cough. I had brought all three patients to the hospital in San Antonio to see my friend, who was one of the best pulmonary doctors in South Texas. He appropriately did a good workup of their coughs, and performed a bronchoscopy on all three women. He found some evidence of inflammation in their upper airways, as I remember, but good cultures of the secretions did not grow any bacteria, yeast, tuberculosis, or other pathogens.

My friend decided these patients had an unusual case of

asthma—without wheezes—and that their only hope was to find an effective cough suppressant. The women all returned to Uvalde in good spirits, knowing they had seen the best doctor available, but were discouraged that no cause for their coughs was found. Because of the relative hopelessness of the diagnosis and their chronicity of symptoms, I decided to give each of them a course of nystatin.

I gave them a couple of pills a day, not really expecting much to change. To my surprise, not just one or two of the women, but all three stopped coughing within a week. I was in disbelief. How could a medicine that does not get in the blood stop a cough in a patient who has no known fungal or bacterial infection in her upper airways? And how could something in the gut cause a chronic cough? Since the only thing I had done was give the patients a nonabsorbable antifungal antibiotic to kill gut yeast, the only plausible answer in my scientific mind was that yeast in the gut somehow caused the chronic cough that molested my patients for so long.

Little did I suspect that this response to therapy in these three little ladies from Uvalde would continue to profoundly influence my medical practice for many years. Suffice it to say the three women remained free of cough for many months. Because I considered the nystatin to be so benign as a medicine, I refilled the nystatin prescriptions for all of them for several months. I had no idea how long they needed to take the nystatin, but I assumed a few months would be enough.

Several months after I stopped prescribing the nystatin, the coughing returned in two of the three women. This time I did not waste money on X-rays or trials of antibacterial antibiotics. I went straight to nystatin tablets twice a day. Again, the cough stopped and continued to cease as long as I kept the patients on nystatin. I finally elected to give them in addition to the nystatin some fluconazole, which I knew had more potential side effects but might kill yeast in the cracks—deep in the valleys and hills of the gut. The results were enlightening. All three women became free of cough after a two-week course of fluconazole, and the cough remained in remission after nystatin and all other medicines were stopped.

As a young physician, I was amazed at this. I was a highly trained internist who had supervised a medical residency program for sixty residents and interns, and I never once heard of yeast causing anything of any importance. I did not blow off the experience but decided I would try the antifungal regimen again in the future when caring for someone who had some other unexplainable disease.

THE LEARNING CURVE

My experience with the three women who had chronic coughs opened my eyes to the possibilities of out-of-the-box thinking. Those women became well because I prescribed treatment that was out of the range of mainstream medicine. As one might imagine, after caring for these people, my mind opened to the possibility that the same therapeutic logic might be useful in other patients who came into my experience.

Over the years, my medical practice became somewhat of a testimony to the veracity of Dr. Crook's suggestion that what grows in your bowel can cause symptoms in a variety of organ systems. I will share with you the stories of three other women—Maria, Rosa, and Emily[5]—all of whom were suffering from the same disease, which I later found out was caused by an overgrowth of yeast. I hope their stories will whet your

---

5   Note that names of all individuals have been changed for this writing.

appetite to learn more about your immune system, appreciate the importance of Dr. Crook's writing, and get a glimpse into what it was like for me as a doctor figuring out the best way to cure something that seemed invisible.

A common disease I've encountered as a nephrologist is systemic lupus erythematosus. This is an autoimmune disease that is usually cared for by internal medicine physicians or rheumatologists when symptoms are mild—but by nephrologists when the condition is bad. Systemic lupus can be mild or severe. In my experience it occurs more often in young women than men and in younger people more often than old. Its common symptoms are rashes of various kinds, diffuse joint pain, muscle fatigue, and pleurisy (painful breathing). When severe, almost all organs, including the heart, brain, and kidneys, become ill. Since people with failing kidneys are placed on dialysis, nephrologists often are blessed to care for young people with systemic lupus. Such was often the case for me.

Systemic lupus is probably the second most commonly seen rheumatologic disease behind rheumatoid arthritis. Patients with lupus often get a facial rash that looks like a red mask particularly involving the forehead and cheeks. The word *lupus* is Latin for "red wolf." Systemic lupus sometimes is a mild disease in which there is a rash or minor aching of joints. Such symptoms are treated with aspirin, ibuprofen, or other relatively tame medicines. Conversely, patients whose kidneys, hearts, and brains are involved are usually quite ill and require aggressive medical therapy. To know what therapy is needed, the cause of the disease needs to be known.

Here is where it gets sticky.

After eighty or more years of research, we still do not know the true cause of systemic lupus. We know a lot about the disease but not its true starting point. Years ago, doctors knew patients with lupus sometimes had significant protein in their urine. Most people have just tiny amounts of protein in the urine—measured in milligrams. Often many grams of protein are in the urine of lupus patients. Sometimes blood cells and other cells are in the urine as well.

When kidneys of sick patients with lupus were biopsied, a very interesting pathologic change was often seen. Stuck on the filter membrane of the several million little filters in the kidneys were millions of tiny protein deposits—like tiny slivers on an otherwise smooth surface. These tiny deposits were found to contain antibodies. The antibodies, however, were not alone. They were attached to minute pieces of DNA from the nuclei of cells. We each have the same DNA in all of our cells, so no one could say the antibodies were stuck onto DNA from the kidneys, brain, heart, or other organs. The only apparent possibility was that the deposits were composed of DNA stuck onto an antibody, or piece of antibody, from somewhere else.

These tiny deposits became known as anti-DNA antibodies, and before long most researchers knew all symptoms of lupus were caused by these deposits circulating all over the body and getting stuck in membranes of diverse tissues. This included the skin with rash, the brain with seizures and encephalopathy, the lungs and pleura with inflammatory reactions (pleuritis, pericarditis, and cardiac arrhythmias), and the kidneys with inflamed basement membranes and loss of kidney function. Lupus became known as an autoimmune disease, with the presumption that antibodies are made against intracellular DNA for some unknown reason and that after this pathologic process gets going, it can be stopped only by disrupting the immune system with drugs.

By the 1970s, we nephrologists were treating our lupus patients with high doses of steroids first and then other anti-immune system drugs like we used to prevent rejections of transplanted organs. The standard cocktail for a sick young woman with lupus became intravenous steroids and Cytoxan (cyclophosphamide) or another transplant drug such as Imuran (azathioprine). The treatment was given repeatedly over many months, as long as the patient had elevated protein in her urine, a bad rash, or evidence of active lupus in some vital organ.

The treatment was nearly as bad as the disease. I am embarrassed to say the treatment of systemic lupus hasn't changed much since 1975. The presumption is that we have no idea why the immune reaction that causes the lupus is active, so the only thing we do is "kill" a portion of the immune system to decrease inflammation that occurs all over the body—especially in the kidneys, heart, joints, and brain. Wouldn't it be cool if someone could find what causes the whole thing to get started in the first place? The answer to this is, of course, yes, but as far as I can read, very little research in progress is designed to get to the cause of lupus. Almost every paper on the subject is devoted to new therapies to disrupt the immune system and therefore prevent organ damage.

MARIA'S STORY

One of the first lupus patients I cared for was a twenty-five-year-old woman I will call Maria—this was in the early 1980s, before I read *The Yeast Connection*. She was a beautiful Hispanic girl, a mother of two young children, with a recurrent rash on her arms and legs and frequent joint pain. Her family doctor referred her to me because she had protein and blood in her urine. Maria had been very healthy until her late teens, when after delivering her first child she began to have muscle and joint pains. Her family doctor told her she probably had a virus, treating her with ibuprofen or a similar medicine. She seemed to get better but thereafter did not feel well much of the time. It was hard enough taking care of a one-year-old, so there was little time to think about ill health.

Eventually, Maria had some blood tests and was found to have anemia. It was presumed this was related to pregnancy and menstrual blood loss, and she was treated with iron supplements. After a couple of years of these symptoms, she developed pleurisy and a cough. Her chest pain was bothersome because it hurt when she breathed. A chest X-ray revealed some fluid below and behind her right lung. With all these symptoms and findings, her doctor suspected something more serious than arthritis and a cold. The blood and protein in her urine indicated kidney disease, so she was referred to my office.

It was kind of a no-brainer to me. I knew this patient had lupus nephritis, and I needed only some blood tests and a kidney biopsy to prove what was wrong with her. I ordered the antibody study for lupus—an antinuclear antibodies (ANA) test. It came back strongly positive in a very high titer, and I told her she had systemic lupus erythematosus and that all her symptoms were because of this disease. She asked me what caused the disease, and I had to tell her no one knew the cause.

I told Maria the disease had been around for one hundred years and that most people who had lupus did pretty well if they took some strong medicines. I knew all about how to give her these medicines. I'm not sure this made her feel a lot better, but I felt proud to be such a good doctor that I could diagnose this unusual disease. I told Maria we would need to do a kidney biopsy so I could better tell her the prognosis for her lupus kidney disease. I'm sure this wasn't very reassuring either, since the biopsy would require her to be in the hospital at least for one night to be sure she didn't develop severe bleeding after the biopsy.

I assured her that most people don't bleed very much after such a biopsy but that we would watch her closely. She may have asked me what the biopsy might show and what the plan would be after we knew its results. I explained that there were at least three different kinds of lupus kidney disease and that all had different prognoses—even with strong medications. In general, the more inflammation present in the kidneys, the stronger the medication we would have to give her to manage her lupus.

Maria underwent the biopsy and thankfully did not have any bleeding or other major complications from the procedure. The biopsy showed the worst kind of lupus kidney disease, which is called rapidly progressive glomerulonephritis with crescents. If we did not very promptly treat her with strong medication, she would shortly be in kidney failure and need dialysis. If this were to happen, I assured her, she would be eligible for a kidney transplant. I'm sure all of this was overwhelming for Maria, but she agreed to move ahead with aggressive therapy.

The following week, she started the standard regimen at that time for treatment of severe lupus nephritis. It consisted of a high dose of prednisone, a form of cortisol. Her other medicine was a drug called Cytoxan (cyclophosphamide), a close cousin to nitrogen mustard, which has been used in chemical warfare weapons—especially during World War I. To treat severe lupus, Cytoxan is given intravenously in very high dosage once a week for five or six weeks. The main side effect of Cytoxan is severely reduced production of red blood cells, white blood cells, and platelets in the bone marrow, resulting in severe anemia and decreased ability to fight off infections. An allied problem with this drug is ulceration of and bleeding from the lining of the urinary bladder.

Cytoxan and steroids (Medrol) both suppress immunity,

making patients vulnerable to infections of all kinds. Maria was frightened about potential side effects, but she bravely received her initial infusions of this chemotherapy for her lupus kidney disease and did very well at first. When I checked the protein in her urine several weeks later, the amount had markedly decreased—indicating to me that she was having a good response to the drugs. Maria went through several cycles of steroids and Cytoxan over the next couple of months, and she seemed to be feeling well with no signs of infection. I was encouraged, as was she.

About three months into her therapy, she called me one day and told me that she felt poorly. She had a low-grade fever, and aching muscles and joints that felt different than her usual lupus symptoms. I told her it was probably a virus. I recommended some aspirin or ibuprofen and advised her to give me a call the next day if she were not feeling a lot better. The next day she felt even worse. Her temperature was over one hundred, and she was developing a rash. I was still thinking it might be a viral illness, but I asked her to come to the clinic so I could take a look at the rash.

She got to the office, and it was clear she was very ill. Her blood pressure was low instead of its usual high, and she appeared pasty, pale, and weak. I didn't know what was wrong with her, but I thought that she needed to be admitted to the hospital. She agreed, and that afternoon, she was admitted to the renal ward. Knowing she was immunosuppressed on her medications, I ordered cultures of her blood and urine as well as usual blood tests routinely done on all new hospital patients. Presuming she might have a kidney infection because of her lupus, I started her on strong antibiotics that had the potential to kill the most common bacteria that might be infecting her blood.

That evening, she became increasingly ill with high fever, chest pain, and even lower blood pressure. I came back to the hospital to see her, and spent a lot of time talking with her husband and her sister. I explained that I was treating her for the most important infections she was likely to have but that the antibiotics hadn't had a chance to work as yet. Late that night, her blood pressure dropped to 30/10, and her pulse became thready and weak. In the midst of this, I received a message from the laboratory that she appeared to have fungus in her blood and signs of severe toxicity in her blood. I ordered a dose of a fairly toxic antifungal drug used commonly at that time.

Unfortunately, Maria's condition deteriorated during the night. She suffered cardiac arrest and could not be resuscitated. I was devastated, and her family was crushed. A young mother had died of apparent fungal sepsis. The source of the fungus was not apparent to me, but in her blood were large numbers of organisms from the family Candida Albicans. This is the same organism Dr. Crook noted to cause all kinds of strange symptoms in multiple organs of the body—not because of fungus in the blood but through the workings of the immune system.

In Maria's case, the yeast was not in her bowel but in her blood. I knew she had experienced an episode of thrush in her mouth several months earlier and vaginal yeast infections on a couple of occasions. But this time, the yeast was not in her vagina or mouth. It had somehow gotten into her blood and killed her—very quickly. I believed in my heart she had gotten the fungus because I gave her strong anti-immune medication to treat her lupus kidney disease. Her decimated immune system lost its ability to effectively kill germs, and some fungus—probably from her bowel or vagina—had somehow escaped into her blood and made her ill. I resolved to not let such a thing happen again.

How wrong I turned out to be! Wanting something to happen or not happen in medicine is not always an easy call. I had a thing or two yet to learn about yeast and immunity.

ROSA'S STORY

The next patient I will tell you about is Rosa. Rosa was in her forties and had been on dialysis in one of my kidney centers for a few years when I met her. She was a good patient and did everything my nurses and I asked her to do. She had gone into renal failure because of lupus, for which she had begun dialysis in another city a number of years before moving to San Antonio. She wanted a kidney transplant, but she had no living donors and was on the cadaver list, waiting for a kidney from someone who lost their life in an accident.

Finally, one evening we received a call from a surgeon who had removed kidneys from a patient killed in an accident in Dallas. The tissue typing center had told him the kidney was a good match for Rosa. He asked if she was in good health, and I assured him Rosa was a very healthy dialysis patient. Arrangements were made, and the kidney was shipped overnight in iced slush solution to San Antonio.

Rosa came to the hospital for emergency dialysis before the transplant. The transplant surgery went beautifully, and by morning, Rosa was urinating normally with a brand-new kidney. We were so happy for her. She was a mother of teenagers, and the family had been waiting for such a long time for Mom to get a new kidney. Her lupus had still been a minor problem over the several years I knew her, but her symptoms were mainly transient rashes and some mild joint pain.

A couple of years earlier, Rosa had experienced a mild case of pericarditis—an inflammation of the sac surrounding the heart.

That condition sometimes occurs in dialysis patients without lupus, so we just dialyzed her more often for a week or so, and the pericarditis resolved. As far as I was concerned, I felt her lupus was not much of a problem at the time of the transplant. Over the next several weeks, Rosa did well and received the usual high doses of medications to suppress her immune system. About three weeks post-transplant, her urine output dropped, and her blood tests showed kidney function was deteriorating. My team and I assumed she was experiencing an acute rejection of the kidney, that her immune system was making chemicals that were killing her transplanted kidney.

We did a kidney biopsy to make sure we knew for sure what was going on, but we also gave her our rescue protocol of high doses of steroids and anti-immune agent OKT-3. Both of these were known to reverse acute rejection of transplanted organs, and Rosa's condition began to get better by about the third day after the new drugs were started. Her kidney function again improved, and we settled into a plan to taper her anti-rejection drugs. Within a couple of weeks, everything was back to the way it was before the rejection.

This sort of thing is fairly common after a transplant, so we continued to hope for a long-term good result. Rosa went home after this event with a bushel load of medications to prevent rejection and to treat her high blood pressure, which had worsened with her rejection episode. Her lupus was the least of the problems, probably because we had given her so much steroids.

All went well for several months, and then we again noticed a falloff in her kidney function. A biopsy of the transplanted kidney again showed acute rejection. I called Rosa and told her she needed to go back in the hospital for another course of intravenous anti-rejection drugs. This occurred over the next several days, and she seemed to do well. Her kidney function stabilized but did not improve much from the level caused by the rejection. We changed her anti-rejection medications somewhat—higher doses of anti-immune therapy—and her kidney function again improved.

About ten days into this therapy, after receiving high doses of steroids and other medications, Rosa developed a fever. We cultured her throat, blood, and urine, and started her on antibiotics. Initially she seemed to improve, but late the following day, her temperature spiked to 103 degrees and her blood pressure dropped.

Although we gave Rosa a truckload of fluids and several good antibiotics, her condition continued to deteriorate over the next twenty-four hours. She suffered first a respiratory arrest and had to be placed on a ventilator, but her health worsened. Too late, we learned one of her blood cultures was growing a fungus. We pulled out our only good medication for treatment of blood fungus, but the drug was too toxic for Rosa, or the sepsis and related poisoning of her blood vessels was too severe. She died late that evening of cardiac arrest as a result of septic shock.

The organism cultured from her blood was—you guessed it—Candida Albicans. The same organism that had killed my other patient, Maria. I was learning that, at least in patients with lupus, the presence of fever in a person receiving anti-immune therapy showed a risk for fungus in the blood.

After becoming acquainted with Dr. Crook's *The Yeast Connection*, I thought more deeply about the connection between lupus and fungus. I cared for many other patients with systemic lupus over the years, and I took care to look for signs of fungus infection. Surprisingly, many had experienced frequent vaginal yeast infections or episodes of thrush in their mouths during their teenage years and beyond. They likely were treated for these with a week or two of nystatin or even a single dosage of fluconazole, which is the current protocol for dealing with such illnesses.

In those days, I did not have the courage to place patients on chronic anti-yeast therapy. It just wasn't the standard of care the healthcare community expected. I could tell you about several such patients, but one stands out for inclusion in this narrative.

EMILY'S STORY

Emily was a seventeen-year-old high school senior referred to my renal clinic for evaluation of protein and blood in her urine. She, like Maria, had a history of vaginal yeast infections—even without her taking antibiotics. When I first saw her, I knew she probably had lupus. Her face was red in the mask pattern of the red wolf. She thought she had acne, but I told her it likely wasn't acne. I explained the characteristics of the rash looking like the markings of a red wolf and tried to explain autoimmune disease. Emily had experienced some joint pain and frequently had a light, slightly raised rash on her forearms and trunk. Her doctors called it a virus or sun poisoning, but she never had a cold, diarrhea, or other signs of viral illness with her rashes.

I measured her twenty-four-hour protein excretion in her urine, and it was quite elevated at around 3.5 grams. The normal is less than 500 mg. Her urine contained lots of red blood cells and some white blood cells, but her urine culture did not reveal any microorganisms. An anti-nuclear antibody test came back strongly positive, and her levels of complement, an inflammatory component, were low—suggesting they had been used up in her daily life. Her blood studies showed mild anemia, which may have been from iron deficiency but that occurs in autoimmune diseases as well.

I felt Emily had lupus erythematosus. I explained to Emily and her mother the same things I had explained to Rosa and Maria about lupus, and what needed to be done to try to stop the disease in its tracks. Emily underwent a renal biopsy, and as expected the kidney filters (glomeruli) were very inflamed in an ugly pattern. We would need to proceed very shortly with aggressive therapy if we hoped to save Emily's kidney function. With some reservation because of Emily's young age, her family gave permission to start her on Cytoxan and high doses of steroids.

By this time, I was somewhat gun-shy because of my previous experiences with giving patients high-dose chemotherapy. I gave Emily a little lower dosage of both medicines, and she seemed to do very well. She was young, strong, and likely had a very functional immune system. Her kidney function seemed to stabilize after her first several infusions of Cytoxan. An episode of bleeding from her bladder required her coming to the hospital to have her bladder washed out with saline. This was sometimes a complication of Cytoxan therapy. A urologist looked into her bladder with a cystoscope and saw many tiny sites of bleeding. He cauterized those with electrolysis, and the bleeding stopped.

Shortly thereafter, Emily's mother called to say that Emily was listless and nauseated. My antennae went up, because I knew she was badly immunosuppressed. I asked her mother to bring her to my office. Her temperature was higher than 101 degrees, and she looked quite ill. She was coughing and breathing rapidly, and I thought she might have pneumonia. I felt Emily needed to be in a hospital for observation.

Thankfully, my instincts made me think beyond the possibility of bacterial pneumonia to unusual infections that occur in immunosuppressed patients. Emily certainly met all the criteria for such a patient. She had lupus, which was of unknown cause, and now she had a very low white blood count and was anemic—because of the medications I'd prescribed. I was scared, because vivid memories of previously similar situations were with me.

Emily was admitted to the hospital that afternoon, and I did the usual cultures of urine, sputum, and blood. I had to decide whether to wait for a positive culture to come back to start antibiotics—or to go ahead with strong antibiotics. I elected to start the antibiotics immediately. This time, however, I treated my patient presumptively with an intravenous antifungal drug, fluconazole, which was relatively newly available from the hospital pharmacy.

During the night, Emily's temperature rose, and her blood pressure dropped. I could feel the third verse of my lupus story pressing down upon me and my beautiful teenage patient. I gave her a bunch of intravenous fluids to try to expand her volume of salt and water, and treat her low blood pressure. By morning, she was surprisingly better. I didn't know which of the medicines was helping, but I didn't give a dang, because she was clearly better. I kept all of the antibiotics and the antifungal drug infusing, and ordered that they be continued for another day, when the results of the blood and urine cultures would be available.

What do you suppose was growing in Emily's blood? Candida Albicans! Emily had four positive blood cultures for Candida. Fortunately, I gave her several doses of fluconazole over that first forty-eight hours in the hospital, and killing the yeast in her blood undoubtedly—in light of my previous experiences—saved her life.

You may be asking by now, like I did, if yeast has anything to do with the underlying cause of systemic lupus. To me, it was a big deal. I began to look for a history of yeast exposure in lupus patients, and it was almost always there. I put some of my patients with lupus and other immunologic diseases on oral nystatin as a prophylactic measure. From my purview, their lupus became more stable in most cases, and their rashes and joint pains were lessened.

I usually didn't have the courage to go out on the line and start fluconazole or another strong systemic antifungal medicine without a good reason to do so. It's one thing to give nystatin, which goes through the gastrointestinal tube without being absorbed. I think patients can, therefore, take nystatin for months or years without side effects. Conversely, any systemic drug—that which is absorbed into the bloodstream from the gut—can cause side effects and must be given with some caution.

Dr. Crook, in his book *The Yeast Connection*, gives a lot of print space to the role of diet in patients who have sensitivity to yeast. I advised all of my patients with lupus to eat an anti-yeast diet per Dr. Crook's instructions.

FROM YEAST TO BACTERIA

It wasn't long before my brain was entering each clinical situation with a new way of looking at patients. I now saw patients not so much as persons having a named disease, which I was proud to know the name of, but rather as people who had processes going on in their bodies—and treatment of the problem was meant to stop the process. I still treated bronchitis patients with antibacterial antibiotics, but I wondered if I should prescribe nystatin at the same time to prevent yeast overgrowth.

Remember, I had no idea whether the problem was too much yeast per square inch of bowel, or something that had changed in the wall of the bowel that caused it to be more sensitive to the usual amount of yeast—as Dr. Crook hypothesized. Forty years later, I still don't know the answer to that question, maybe because both situations prevail in varying patients. Suffice it to say I tried the nystatin regimen on a number of patients for a variety of symptoms in a variety of parts of the body. Amazingly, many improved or had symptoms disappear altogether.

I remember thinking also that if yeast organisms in the gut can induce an immune reaction that causes symptoms in distant organs, then bacteria in the gut could likely do the same. In this sense, I took a step away from Dr. Crook's hypothesis that weird stuff happens only because of immune reactions to yeast. I read papers on the gut and its bacteria, and I couldn't find anything about gut bacteria causing any disease.

My instincts told me my hypothesis about gut bacteria was correct—it did have an effect similar to that of yeast on the immune system. But if bacteria—not yeast—were the root cause of certain illnesses, then the solution was a lot more complicated. The treatment I had been giving for yeast was nystatin, which had almost no risk of side effects thanks to its nonabsorbability into the blood. The same cannot be said for antibiotics, which are used to treat bacteria.

Before exploring the relationship between gut bacteria and disease, let's look at what we know about bacteria in the body and the dangers of antibiotics.

CHAPTER SEVEN

UNDERSTANDING THE BACTERIA IN OUR BODIES

More than one thousand species of microorganisms grow along the tube. Some are yeasts. Some are bacteria. Some are protozoans. Each of the thousand or so species has specific physical, biochemical, and physiologic characteristics. They are of different sizes and shapes, and have appetites for different kinds of foods—just like humans. They make chemicals and release them into their surrounding environment. Some of these chemicals are poison to their neighbors. This must be how they keep unwanted neighbors from entering their territory. Some require oxygen to live and flourish. Others can't live when oxygen is present. They live in what is called biofilm.

The biofilm is a mucous membrane of various thickness that lines the entire bowel from the mouth to the anus. It is full of microorganisms and acts as a covering for other germs growing between the mucous layer and the bowel. Think of it as a rich covering made of microorganisms, nutrients, and dissolved food products. The latter come from us. We eat a variety of nutrients that together determine to some extent how well the various kinds of microorganisms live and thrive. What we eat is likely very important in this regard. It doesn't take much ingenuity to suggest that food exerts its effects on human health, not so much by the effect of the nutrients absorbed into the cellular apparatus, but by the effect of food on microflora in a person's biome.

In the past ten to fifteen years, this information has become common knowledge, and more books have been written about the biome than in any other time in history.[6] I was exploring these topics long before it was discovered that gut microorganisms have any impact at all on health—before it was found that duodenal and gastric peptic ulcers are mostly caused by gut bacteria, specifically a gut inhabitant called *Helicobacter pylori*. I grew up in a time when we were taught that ulcers were brought on by too much acid in the stomach and stressful life issues—not by bacteria. In fact, famous gastroenterologists were on record saying there could be no bacteria in the stomach because all germs would die in the stomach's acid.

This was the dogma all gastroenterology fellows were taught until the late 1980s, when some doctors from Australia discovered that scraping away the coat of mucous that lines the stomach revealed that the area under the mucous was often loaded with a number of species of bacteria. I suspect some yeast organisms were there as well. It was determined over the next couple of decades that helicobacter organisms caused

---

6   Books on the topic include *Grain Brain: The Surprising Truth about Wheat, Carbs, and Sugar—Your Brain's Silent Killers* and *Brain Maker: The Power of Microbes to Heal and Protect Your Brain for Life* by Dr. David Perlmutter; *The Good Gut: Taking Control of Your Weight, Your Mood and Your Long-term Health* by Justin and Erica Sonnenburg; *The End of Alzheimer's: The First Program to Prevent and Reverse Cognitive Decline* by Dr. Dale E. Bredesen; and a number of other titles by various authors.

not only peptic ulcers but also lymphomas of the bowel and a number of other chronic illnesses.

At the time, I felt I had been lied to by professors who said no bacteria were in the upper bowel. They were wrong, and therapy for ulcers—which often included a surgical procedure called vagotomy and pyloroplasty—changed dramatically. It's hard forty years later to find a general surgical colleague who has ever performed a vagotomy and pyloroplasty procedure. I remember thinking we really didn't know diddly-squat about the organisms in the gut, that there was a lot to learn about them, and that a lot of diseases were probably related to what I had observed in my dialysis patients.

This thinking, and the positive experiences of treating some patients with nystatin, helped me see outside dogmatic academic thought. I wondered if bacteria might in fact have a similar impact on the immune system as yeast did.

About one thousand different species of bacteria grow on the surface of the large and small bowels. They represent a far greater percentage of total organisms than do candida and other yeast. I would guess that normal yeast levels in the bowel one hundred years ago were in 1 percent to 2 percent of organisms.

In the past fifty years, the use of antibiotics, disinfectants, and pesticides has changed the flora so that now a larger percentage of yeast and somewhat smaller percentage of bacteria grow in our bowels. This may be one reason yeast is an increasingly common cause of strange immunologic phenomena. Our grandparents were exposed to far lower percentages of yeast in the bowel than our present generations. Nevertheless, the vast majority of microorganisms growing in our bowels have always been bacteria. They have now been studied extensively, and the DNA sequences of many are known.

If bacteria grow more abundantly in our bowels than yeast,

wouldn't it stand to reason that bacteria cause similar sorts of reactions as yeast—and could cause numerous previously unexplained illnesses? But settling on bacteria as a cause, especially when there were no tests to prove it, was riskier than following treatments for yeast. This is largely because of the lesser impact in treating yeast.

THE DANGERS OF ANTIBIOTICS

Because nystatin isn't absorbed into the blood, it is a relatively safe drug to prescribe for a long period of time. The same cannot be said for antibiotics, which are used to treat bacteria. What dangers can follow the use of antibiotics? A number of risks exist, but I will focus on the few I consider to be most important.

First of all, note that there are at least seven general classes of antibiotics—each kills specific germs more or less effectively than the others. Any of these drugs in any class can cause a severe allergic reaction or even death because of anaphylactic shock, which is the inability to maintain blood pressure. The same drugs in selected individuals can cause rashes, kidney and liver diseases, joint pains, cardiac arrhythmias, and a host of other symptoms. Any physician who prescribes an antibiotic lives with the possibility that the medicine could cause a bad allergic reaction.

Second, almost every antibiotic known to man can kill normal bacteria growing in the tube. With upward of a thousand species of organisms growing in the intestinal tubes, any or many are vulnerable to damage and death when exposed to the antibiotics used to treat bronchitis, otitis, and urinary tract infections. This is precisely what happens and leads to the overgrowth of yeast in the mouth, rectum, and vagina when certain antibiotics are used to treat other illness. It seems unlikely Dr. Crook would have written *The Yeast Connection* had he not seen patients given antibiotics for treatment of other infections—thus resulting in yeast infections.

Let's look at this in more detail. Sometimes antibiotic treatment of one type of bacterial infection leads to overgrowth of other more toxic bacteria, which make their own toxins and cause disease. A classic case of this phenomenon occurs when Clostridium difficile organisms grow luxuriantly in the bowels of those treated with ampicillin for bronchitis. The diarrhea and abdominal cramping the C. difficile causes is far more debilitating than the bronchitis. Stronger antibiotics of another type entirely are needed to kill the C. difficile. Allergic reactions, and growth of yeast and unwanted bacteria, are the most important complications of antibacterial antibiotics used for treatment of minor illnesses that might not even be caused by bacteria in the first place.

Another even more insidious complication of antibiotic use is on the minds and hearts of doctors. As is common knowledge, the widespread use of antibiotics has led to the development of antibiotic resistance. Germs formerly killed by penicillin now survive and enjoy a good meal when exposed to penicillin. The bacteria, over a period of time, learned to make chemicals that inactivate the antibiotics.

This happens in nature all the time. Fungi make chemicals like penicillin that kill bacteria. Bacteria make toxins like fluconazole that inactivate fungi. There is apparently a learning curve for all microorganisms as they learn to deal with their neighbors and the toxins their neighbors construct to protect their offspring. Antibiotic resistance has become a difficult problem—particularly in hospitals where patients have received very strong antibiotics for treatment of difficult infections.

A chief benefactor of this antibiotic resistance syndrome is methicillin-resistant staphylococcus (MRSA), an organism that was unheard of in the 1960s, when penicillin was used to kill almost every kind of bacteria. Penicillin was especially successful in killing staphylococcus, which was our most common skin organism. The intravenous version of penicillin, Methicillin, killed all staph organisms. This antibiotic was a close cousin of penicillin, used very successfully around the world.

Unfortunately, by the late 1970s, a number of staph organisms were found in hospital laboratories to be less effectively killed by previously very effective antibiotics. The organisms being tested from hospitalized patients could no longer be killed with Methicillin. This obviously caused a lot of problems for us doctors who were taking care of very sick people in the hospital. After that time, we could not just assume Methicillin would kill the staph which was causing a skin or wound infection. We had to do special cultures and use antibiotics that were more toxic in order to kill germs that previously died quickly when exposed to Methicillin.

This resistance syndrome has occurred with many antibiotics, so that at present, many bacteria show a great deal of resistance to commonly used antibiotics of all kinds. Researchers continue to look for and develop new antibiotics that are more effective at killing the old germs than were the antibiotics used commonly in the previous century. Hopefully this pattern continues, and we will always have at our disposal good antibiotics capable of killing whatever is causing infection in our patients.

THE PHYSICIAN'S DILEMMA

Obviously, millions of people all over the world are treated annually with antibacterial antibiotics for pulmonary infections, bronchitis, urinary tract infections, colon infections, ear infections, and so on. There is no argument from anyone about the tremendous value of antibiotics in this setting—they have saved millions of lives each year.

There is an almost constant dialogue between academic medicine and the general public, however, about the dangers of antibiotics used to treat diseases that are not bacterial. For instance, ample evidence shows that the great majority of people who have viral upper respiratory illnesses do not need to be treated with antibiotics. Viruses do not respond to antibiotics, and in most cases the immune system steps up and destroys the virus after a few hours, days, or weeks. Academic physicians are quick to point this out to those of us who are taking care of sick people down in the pits.

The same physicians know that most people don't get damaged too badly by a virus—when people get sick, it's often because of bacterial secondary infection of tissues injured by the virus. The virus does initial damage to tissues of the lungs, bronchi, ears, throat, skin, or other location. This is followed on occasion by invasion of bacteria that normally live in the area—like streptococcus, staphylococcus, or pseudomonas. We doctors are supposed to become adept at telling whether a patient has a simple viral infection or if the viral infection is complicated by invasion of a bacterium. This is so important because bacterial otitis, bronchitis, sinusitis, meningitis, and pneumonia are very serious problems. These medical problems often do not get better quickly or later result in serious secondary illnesses and complications such as chronic pleural infection, chronic sinus infection, chronic otitis, cellulitis of the skin, and other serious infections.

Physicians are in a constant state of worrying about whether or not an illness is bacterial. There are telltale signs of bacterial invasion, but they are not always easy to see. Many patients have become far more ill than they should have because of a delayed treatment for bacterial illness, which further complicated a viral invasion of tissues. Patients know this and often remember times they received antibiotics and got better very quickly. Nevertheless, doctors have to constantly tell patients they likely do not need antibiotics for illnesses that present with classic viral symptoms.

In truth, many primary care physicians and medical subspecialists prescribe antibiotics liberally to patients who have unclear diagnoses. This angers academic infectious disease experts, who have been stating for years that antibiotics can cause all kinds of problems when overused or used to treat diseases not caused by bacteria.

This creates challenges for primary care physicians to be good at what they do. If they hold to the academic line and don't use antibiotics until they are sure of a bacterial problem, they are likely to see some patients become very sick because of the delay in treating the illness. If they prescribe antibiotics to everyone who has a common cold, their peers and those in academic medicine will criticize them for overuse of antibiotics and the dangers that follow.

This is partly the dilemma I faced when I started hypothesizing that antibiotics could cure unknown diseases by killing gut-dwelling bacteria that was affecting the immune system. But as my patient Bill would show, the results would be worth it.

CHAPTER EIGHT

TACKLING THE BACTERIA WITHIN US

n my obesity clinic, in the 1990s, was a patient who was an educator in a local business, and he successfully lost more than eighty pounds on a very low-calorie diet at the institution. Afterward, he entered a maintenance program, coming in once a month to recheck his weight and blood pressure, and to be accountable for good behavior relative to his body composition.

Sometime in the mid-1990s, this patient—let's call him Bill—went to Mexico and came back to San Antonio with severe diarrhea. This is not uncommon, because the normal bacterial flora of those living in Mexico is significantly different than that in colons of United States' residents. E. coli organisms, for example, are of different species and subtypes. Common bowel organisms vary somewhat in species and immune specificity in different locales and often cause disease in those who are traveling from their homes to new locations. When Americans go to Mexico, they may become quite ill with enteric illness even if they "don't drink the water." Local food can cause problems, even if bottled water is consumed during travel.

Such was the case for Bill, who took a little trip down to Mexico (to quote the Kingston Trio). Bill's diarrhea was treated with antispasmodic drugs and perhaps some Pepto Bismol. Within a week of his return, he noticed rather diffuse joint pain in his wrists, elbows, shoulders, hips, knees, and ankles. The pain was severe, and he had great difficulty driving to work and doing simple daily activities. These symptoms continued even after the diarrhea had gone away.

I did some blood tests that determined Bill had rheumatoid arthritis. He had suffered from obesity and a number of minor problems in the past, but on this occasion, he was quite ill with acute arthritis of multiple symmetric joints. Not knowing anything else to do, I gave him a steroid dose pack, and his joints improved very quickly. Nevertheless, within a couple of days of stopping the steroids, his joint pain returned with a vengeance. For some reason, I felt the problem was unlikely to be related to a fungus in his bowel, but that because he had come back from Mexico with diarrhea, the joint pain was more likely related to bacteria.

This was an intellectual stretch, but it seemed logical the diarrhea—even though it had dissipated—had something to do with the joint pain. I guess I remembered the story of the strep bacteria causing allergic inflammatory kidney disease and all the patients with heart valve infections who had suffered with arthritis.

At any rate, I hypothesized that Bill had some kind of immune problem that started in his bowel and now caused severe cartilage inflammation—best characterized as rheumatoid arthritis. I really didn't know what to do for him. Bill was obviously very ill, and I guess I could have referred him to one of my rheumatology buddies. In those days, rheumatologists treated rheumatoid arthritis with injections of gold, aspirin, and steroids. The nonsteroidal medicines like ibuprofen were just hitting the market, but in truth, there was no good permanent therapy for rheumatoid arthritis.

I knew this, and I liked Bill, and he didn't want another set of doctors involved in his care. Deep in my heart and mind was a desire to give him nystatin and see what happened. I was plagued, however, with this nagging sensation that Bill's problem was not likely related to yeast in the bowel. He was perfectly well until he went to Mexico, where he ate or drank something that caused his diarrhea. I had checked his stools for salmonella and shigella, two common bacteria that can cause severe diarrhea, and Bill's cultures were negative for these as well as a common form of E. coli seen south of the border. I nevertheless had a hunch that bacteria rather than yeast had something to do with his diarrhea and the rheumatoid disease.

This sent me on a search for literature on the subject of causes for rheumatoid arthritis. I already knew the cause was unknown, but I assumed someone somewhere had written about plausible potential causes. I went straight to that era's bible of rheumatology: a massive tome titled *Arthritis and Allied Conditions: A Textbook of Rheumatology* by Joseph Lee Hollander. My reading over the next day or two on rheumatoid arthritis was exciting. In the 1950s and 1960s, quite a few good scientific papers were written on the possible causes of rheumatoid arthritis, or RA for short.

In general, the causes fell into two camps. One group of professors believed rheumatoid arthritis was caused by a previously present episode of gonorrhea. The other group had seen lots of RA patients who had never experienced gonorrhea. Heated arguments on the subject erupted among groups of good physicians. Clearly lots of people who had chronic gonorrhea later developed RA. And probably equal or larger number of individuals who never had this venereal disease nevertheless developed symmetric joint pain. After the disease got going, it was often chronic and led to progressive destruction of the joints—all over the body.

Professors who attested that the disease was not caused by gonorrhea ultimately won the argument, and today—fifty years later—we still do not know the cause of rheumatoid arthritis. This group of academics won the argument because indeed a lot of people with RA never had gonorrhea. Nevertheless, Hollander's textbook and case reports in the medical literature profiled people who had rheumatoid arthritis and got better after taking antibiotics. The problem was that when the antibiotics were stopped, the joint pain usually returned in all its fury.

Also, some papers in the rheumatoid arthritis literature suggested changes in diet could influence a degree of joint pain in RA patients. The results of dietary modification were almost never permanent and did not cure the disease. Nevertheless, there was an inference that germs or food in the gut could influence the severity and course of rheumatoid disease.

With this knowledge, I discussed with Bill our options for therapy of his rheumatoid disease. We knew we could get the joint pain to go away with steroids, but that this was not a good long-term therapy because of side effects. I hypothesized that the best chance for a cure—if bacteria in his bowel had anything whatsoever to do with his diarrhea and joint pain—was a long course of antibiotics to kill the offending bacteria (or bacteria and yeast). Bill agreed to a course of antibiotics along with another short course of steroids to shut off the joint pain.

Bill and I prayed together and began the therapy. Bill took a Medrol Dosepak for the next five days and at the same time began Cipro, which is the antibiotic most used in the treatment of traveler's diarrhea. As expected, the Medrol immediately made his joints better. He was able to drive and do all normal activities. He had no trouble taking the Cipro twice a day, and he continued to have generally normal bowel activity. Unfortunately, as he got to the last day of the steroids in low dose, he again felt his joints beginning to hurt. He continued to take the Cipro as ordered, twice daily, but within three or four days of stopping the steroids, his diffuse joint pain returned with a vengeance.

I was discouraged. My idea that bacteria had something to do with his rheumatoid arthritis was clearly wrong—or I hadn't used the right antibiotic or correct dosage. I told him I could refer him to a rheumatologist, who might be able to help him.

To my surprise, Bill insisted we try again with a different antibiotic. Somewhat reluctantly, I agreed but told him I was not confident that another antibiotic would give a better result—I believed Cipro to be an excellent antibiotic for killing colon bacteria. I still do thirty years later. We decided on cephalexin as the next antibiotic. This is the antibiotic I usually prescribe to treat mouth, skin, or upper respiratory infections. Bill started back on another Medrol Dosepak, which he liked because he knew he'd get a few days of pain relief while taking the steroids. He began taking 250 mg of cephalexin (Keflex) four times per day—a dosage I would recommend for an upper respiratory infection with bacterial bronchitis.

As expected, the steroids worked again, and Bill became free of all joint pain by the third day of the Dosepak. He tolerated the cephalexin well and had normal bowel activity. This time he continued for a few days to have only mild joint pain after stopping the steroids but continuing on the cephalexin. Within a week, however, Bill's pain recurred with its usual intensity.

He was miserable and nearly incapacitated. I told him I had done everything I could and that my idea regarding the cause of rheumatoid arthritis was clearly off base.

Bill again begged for one more trial of a different antibiotic. I told him I was running out of ideas but then remembered a few case reports of rheumatoid disease being improved with tetracycline. This old-time antibiotic has been added to animal feeds since the early 1950s and used to treat teen acne. I told Bill I was willing to give it a try but obviously wasn't very confident it would work any better than Cipro or cephalexin.

We began as usual with another Medrol Dosepak, which was clearly very consistent in making his joint pain disappear. He started the tetracycline at 250 mg four times per day, which was the dosage recommended for treatment of several types of infection. Bill finished the Medrol pack five days later with joints not hurting. He felt remarkably well by that time, but we weren't surprised—this was exactly what had happened on the previous tries. This time, however, Bill's joint pain did not recur as he finished the steroids. I was amazed. I kept waiting for him to call and tell me his rheumatoid symptoms were returning stronger than ever. The call never came. A week went by, then two weeks and three—no joint pain! His bowel activity was normal, and he had no joint pain even after discontinuing the steroids.

After a month of feeling perfectly well, Bill asked me if he was cured of rheumatoid arthritis. I told him I didn't know, but that he may indeed be so. We both rejoiced and thanked the Lord we had found something that reversed the process of what he picked up in Mexico. Bill asked me if he should stop the tetracycline. I had no reason to tell him no. He stopped the antibiotic after four weeks of therapy. A week later Bill called. The joint pain had recurred and was stronger than ever.

He asked if he could go back on the tetracycline and steroids. I agreed and told him that this time we would keep the tetracycline going for a longer period of time. He started another Medrol Dosepak to make his joints well and restarted the tetracycline at the same dose as before. Again, he felt well, and after stopping the steroids, he continued to be free of joint pain. I was thrilled and wondered what germ we had been treating with the antibiotic. I told him to take the tetracycline for about three months before stopping to see whether his joint pain might recur.

Bill remained free of joint pain as long as he was taking the tetracycline. I was comfortable with his taking the antibiotic for this long period of time, because I knew many adults who had taken tetracycline for several years at a time when they had teenage acne. Bill continued the antibiotic regime for three months. I began to give him nystatin twice a day, because I didn't want him to get a yeast-mediated disease from taking the antibiotic for an extended time. After three months free of joint pain, I told him he was likely cured of the rheumatoid disease. I felt he could safely stop the tetracycline.

He did so and remained free of joint pain for about a month. Slowly but surely, he again developed pain in his joints. We were both dumbfounded. We had stumbled by hook or crook into finding out how to make his joint pain go away. What we did not know was how long he would need to take the tetracycline to be absolutely well. We tried another round of the same therapy, having him take the tetracycline for six months. He felt wonderful and stopped the antibiotics again after six months. About a month after stopping, the joint pain returned, again.

I was very surprised at this because we doctors believe in giving antibiotics for ten to fourteen days for most illnesses, and this appears to be sufficient. In this case, we had identified a chronic disease that went away only when we turned off the inflammatory process with steroids and continued with antibiotics chronically. We decided to give the antibiotics one more try—this time even longer. For the following year, Bill took tetracycline four times per day with the accompanying nystatin. He continued this regimen for the entire year and then stopped the tetracycline.

Amazingly, his joint pain never recurred. That was more than twenty-five years ago. He continued to take the nystatin, but he never again needed to take an antibiotic for prevention of joint pain. Many patients have other complications of rheumatoid arthritis, such as rashes, nerve pain, Raynaud's phenomenon, and inflamed arteries. Bill has had none of these. In my mind and his, we believe he had an episode of rheumatoid arthritis that was somehow reversed with his taking antibiotics for a year.

LEARNING FROM BILL'S STORY

I often pondered why Bill's medication needed to be taken for such a long time. The only answer that kept coming to me was that Bill had experienced some change in the bacterial flora of his bowel and the change was exceedingly difficult to eradicate. The bacterial organisms in the bowel wall had induced Bill's immune system to make chemicals that caused acute severe cartilage inflammation far from the bowel. The immune chemical—whatever it was—could be turned off with a Medrol Dosepak, but the minute the steroids were not present, production of the immune system chemicals resumed—at least as long as any of the new bacteria obtained in Mexico were present in Bill's bowel.

ROLE OF STEROIDS IN TREATMENT

Because they don't seem to go away with antibiotics, most diseases of unknown cause are presumed not to be infectious. My opinion in this arena is that the symptoms of the immune-mediated disease are often so severe that initiating antibiotic or antifungal therapy alone would often make us think bacteria and fungus are not involved in the disease process.

Antibiotics or antifungal agents given alone are often not strong enough to shut off an overactive immune response to the organisms. Thus, use of antibiotics alone—without concomitant use of steroids—would often be presumed to be of no benefit to the patient. Sometimes, the medicines need to be used together.

I often take the position that, to reduce symptoms, it is reasonable to turn off the immune system with a short course of steroids at the beginning of antimicrobial therapy—and then see if antimicrobial therapy maintains symptom remission induced at the front door with steroids.

With Bill, who was treated with tetracycline for many months, I would have never known antibiotics would help him if I hadn't first gotten rid of most of his symptoms with steroids. Steroids, which are normal production items in our bodies—and made by our immune systems—may need to be used to get rid of symptoms before the true cause of a disease can be ascertained.

Short courses of Medrol and prednisone are relatively harmless in the long term, but they sometimes help us learn whether symptoms of some terrible disease can go into remission when the immune system is suppressed. Of course, steroids are not the cure, and it's important to keep that in mind. Short courses of steroids make allergies better transiently and may alleviate pain from a distant injury, but that's it. Long-term use of steroids is clearly toxic and is not the answer to the treatment of many diseases.

Doctors have not been taught how much antibiotic is necessary to change the organisms growing in the wall of the large or small intestine. Instead, we were taught that most infections can be treated successfully with antibiotics for ten to fourteen days. Difficult infections like those on heart valves may need longer antibiotic therapy in the range of six to eight weeks to kill off present organisms. Bowel wall organisms, however, are apparently quite different to treat than the same organisms invading the skin or upper airways. We don't know *why* a bowel wall germ can be harder to treat than the same germ living on the surface of the skin, but numerous research groups around the world are attempting to answer that question.

It was clear that longer-term antibiotics, far from being dangerous, had been good for Bill and gave him a new lease on life. We managed to tackle the source of the problem—the foreign bacteria—instead of simply treating symptoms, and it made all the difference.

Let's look at another case study in which long-term antibiotics directed toward healing bacteria in the gut helped a person suffering from an illness.

DAN'S STORY

Dan came to me at the request of his wife, who was a patient. Dan was a middle-aged engineer who had been in generally good health until five years earlier, when he developed high blood pressure. He was placed on a couple of blood pressure medications, which had apparently been reasonably effective in managing his pressures. The fact that he required two drugs to control his blood pressure told me it was significantly high.

His wife, however, did not ask me to see him about his blood pressure. She told me he had recently developed significant muscular weakness and some joint pain. His rheumatology specialist told him he had a disease known as polymyalgia rheumatica. I knew this to be a sometimes devastating disease of the elderly and that it could lead to sudden blindness because of inflammation of the retinal arteries.

Dan did not have any vision problems, but he obviously was quite debilitated from his illness. His rheumatologist had rightly given him a course of steroids to turn off his immune system, since polymyalgia rheumatica is known to be an immunologic illness. Dan got better as expected with the steroids, but unfortunately, as the steroids were tapered, his symptoms again worsened. He was having trouble getting out of bed and had to stop working for a while—a little like Bill with the rheumatoid arthritis. Dan's rheumatologist suggested one of several strong drugs available for treatment of immune diseases—likely methotrexate, hydroxychloroquine, or Imuran (azathioprine)—while increasing his steroids back to a higher level.

At this point, his wife called and asked if I would give them some advice. I think she had heard me speak of immunologic disease in a wellness talk I gave at our church. I met with Dan and his wife, and after listening to the story, began a discussion of bacterial or yeast influence on the initiation of some immunologic diseases. They were anxious to try anything other than the immune-suppressant drugs. In this setting, I felt comfortable trying either an antifungal or antibacterial approach—or both—coupled with a short course of higher-dose steroids to turn off the current immune inflammation of his muscles and nerves.

Because of my experience treating Bill's rheumatoid arthritis, I elected to start Dan on doxycycline, nystatin, and steroids. The latter made his muscles stronger and less painful, and we were hopeful the addition of the antibiotic and antifungal agent would somehow get to the root of what was causing his illness.

As we tapered the steroids, Dan was well for a few days, but then his symptoms recurred with a vengeance. I was so disappointed. I told Dan and his wife that polymyalgia rheumatica must have some different etiology and was obviously not caused by any microorganisms that were treatable with doxycycline. To my surprise, they asked if I would try a different antibiotic. I told them there are a half dozen different classes of antibiotics that kill bacteria of various kinds but that I doubted any would do much better than the doxycycline. I agreed, however, to write a prescription for an antibiotic that killed a slightly different group of bacteria.

This time, I chose cephalexin, an older cephalosporin antibiotic I typically use to treat skin infections, dental problems, and some upper respiratory illnesses. We continued the nystatin to protect against the growth of yeast while he was taking the antibiotic. We also started the steroids back up with a Medrol Dosepak. Dan's muscle weakness improved on the steroids, and he tolerated the antibiotic well. Amazingly, as he tapered off the steroids—but continued with the cephalexin and nystatin—his muscle weakness and pain did not return. I waited expectantly, calling him and his wife each day during the next two weeks to check on his condition.

Dan's muscle weakness never again returned. He remained off the steroids and has never needed them again. He asked me how long he should take the cephalexin, and I told him—based upon my experience with Bill's rheumatoid arthritis—that he might need to take the antibiotic for a long time, perhaps months. He said he felt better than he had for a long time and that he was experiencing no adverse effects whatsoever from the antibiotic. I told him to continue with the nystatin to make sure he did not develop any yeast-related issues. Dan agreed.

I called Dan often, mostly because I could not believe his

disease had disappeared. We had prayed together before we began the therapy, so I was willing to acknowledge this as a spiritual miracle. Additionally, the most amazing thing happened over the next few weeks. Dan noticed his blood pressure getting lower with each passing week, and he was getting a little dizzy whenever he rose from a sitting position. I checked Dan's blood pressure, which was only 90/60. That's pretty low for a guy who supposedly had high blood pressure and was on two drugs for it. We stopped one and then the other of his medications, and his pressure never rose again above 120/70. Dan had not lost weight nor changed anything else about his routine. He told me that somehow the antibiotic had corrected whatever was causing his elevated blood pressure.

As a busy nephrologist taking care of patients with terribly high blood pressure—often on four or five drugs with moderate control—I was amazed. Never in my dreams would I have considered prescribing an antibiotic regimen to lower someone's blood pressure. In Dan's case, however, that is exactly what happened, and his pressures remained normal. As he passed by one year on the low dose of cephalexin and nystatin, he told me he saw no reason for stopping either medication. He felt well, had normal bowel activity, was energetic and going to work each day, and had no symptoms whatsoever of polymyalgia rheumatica.

At the time of this writing, five years have passed, and Dan still takes a low dose of cephalexin and his usual nystatin. His blood pressure averages 125/75 with no blood pressure medications. I am amazed. Nothing in my medical literature suggests bacteria have anything to do with blood pressure control. Then again, I had never before treated someone with high blood pressure with long-term antibiotics. Perhaps someone else will try it, or maybe I will have the courage to try it with other patients.

CHANGING THE BACTERIA WITHIN US

Bill and Dan's stories prove that antibiotics can impact microflora in the gut, but it takes a much longer course than the usual ten to fourteen days. Given the negatives of antibiotics, this is not ideal but sometimes necessary to ensure a patient's overall health.

Some people change the biome in their gut with dietary measures, not antibiotics, although the treatment isn't precise. One of the first examples of someone changing the microorganisms in his gut comes from *The Maker's Diet: The 40-day Health Experience that Will Change Your Life Forever*, a book written by Jordan S. Rubin.

The Maker's Diet is mostly about Rubin's own trials and tribulations. As a very young man, he had severe diarrhea of unknown cause. He, therefore, presented to his physicians much like my patient Bill who had rheumatoid arthritis. Rubin's diarrhea, however, did not get better with Cipro, ampicillin, tetracycline, or other common antibiotics. Rubin sought out the best physicians in his community and was diagnosed with a severe case of an inflammatory bowel disease known as Crohn's disease. Of unknown cause, the disease is associated with weight loss, bloody diarrhea, development of bowel obstructions, and dangerous fistulas between loops of the small intestine.

Rubin began his journey with Crohn's disease at a weight of more than two hundred pounds and a height of more than six feet. After several years of failed medical management of his disease, he was chronically ill and down to around 120 pounds. He and his mother travelled all over the globe to receive various kinds of therapies from world-renowned physicians in many countries. He failed to get well with the standard therapy for Crohn's disease in the United States—some combination of steroids and various immune-suppressant medications. But nothing worked very well for Rubin, and he was moving rapidly toward death from his disease.

I may not have the story exactly right, but when he was hovering near death's doorstep, his father, who was a medical practitioner, I believe, visited a resort in Canada and was told about the healing power of herbs and plants in the region. He obtained some of this local medicine and was given what appeared to be a jar of dirt—that's right, moist black dirt. It was a simple soil sample from a remote area not frequented by people. The dirt was sent to his son, who ingested a few teaspoons dissolved in water. I'm sure it tasted terrible, but almost immediately, Jordin Rubin began to feel better. He continued ingesting the dirt, and within a short time, his diarrhea stopped. Joint pain, skin rash, and other symptoms disappeared, and he regained his weight.

As I remember, no one knew for sure what was in the dirt, but it didn't matter because the patient was getting well. Over time, Rubin returned to over two hundred pounds. He became a fit athlete and wrote a book about his experiences. He adopted a "back to earth" or "back to heaven" diet, believing the secret to good health lies in a diversity of organic vegetables and fruits. His book sold millions of copies, and I'm sure he gained much notoriety and helped a lot of people who were eating unhealthfully.

From my perspective, I saw only proof that dirt from Canada can cure severe Crohn's disease. I have little doubt the dirt contained thousands of microorganisms that had never seen the inside of a human bowel and were capable of changing Rubin's bowel flora by killing microorganisms that were in essence killing him. I have not heard much of Rubin's book in recent years, but the teaching point is clear: changing the flora of the bowel can do amazing things in modifying how the immune system does its work—probably able to contribute to both the good and bad of immunity.

In the past couple of decades, a great amount of research has been undertaken in the realm of so-called fecal transplantation. This is a procedure in which patients with stubborn cases of Crohn's disease, ulcerative colitis, and other enteric diseases have the colon secretions of healthy individuals injected, and thus transplanted, into their colons. Amazingly, a large number of diseases, as well as severe bacterial overgrowth syndromes, have been successfully treated in this manner.

The healthy bacteria of one person are apparently able to establish a beachhead in the colon of another human being, and a new hybrid biome has been created. That this leads to an improvement in health of the recipient is most remarkable and demonstrates that a huge variety of illnesses are in some way related to the organisms that grow in the colon—and how those organisms relate to immune system activity. I suspect that during the next several decades, fecal transplants will be used to treat a variety of diseases of unknown cause.

I recently heard that a world-class female cyclist underwent a fecal transplant from the bowel of another woman who had consistently better bicycle performance in world cyclic events. I know this is hard to believe, but the recipient apparently had a significant improvement in her cycling times and endurance after completion of the fecal transplant. It's amazing what some human beings will do to gain a competitive advantage. The point is that what grows in the bowels influences health in ways we cannot possibly imagine. The jury is still out as to how many diseases can be successfully treated with fecal transplants, but it is an important area in medical research.

This brings us to a discussion of how difficult it is to change the bacterial and fungal colonization of membranes and thus the influence of the biome on the immune system. At the present time, not many good studies are available to answer this question. We know from pretty good studies that the biome of the bowel is pretty well established by age three, so from a microorganism standpoint, we are who we are from early childhood. We know that caesarian section influences the content of the newborn's biome. We know that children who received breast milk have a different biome content than those who did not.

Finally, we know that farm children and others who play in the dirt and around cow poop have a different and more diverse biome than do those who grow up in sterile environments. We know the latter group of children have more allergic events, asthma, and skin conditions like eczema than do children raised in rural or agricultural environments. We know we can change the biome—at least transiently with antibiotics. We know transplants of fecal material from one individual to another can dramatically change the course of a number of diseases by changing the biome.

What we don't know is how long we need to take an antibiotic to permanently change the biome. Based upon the data reported, we also don't know how long we have to take antibiotics or antifungal agents to affect change in disease states. We simply know from the work of Dr. Crook and others that killing germs can sometimes profoundly change the course of diseases that seemingly have nothing to do with germs—at least not at the present.

It remains possible that microorganisms are the starting point for all that goes wrong in the human body. When we learn to control the microorganisms and their role in chronic disease, we in the medical community will likely be much more successful in management of chronic health problems that plague society at present.

I go on record in stating that I have believed for the past several decades that the complex flora of the bowel is integrally involved in the pathogenesis of most chronic diseases. Amazingly, we know surprisingly little about this association, and there are reasons for this. Remember that as recently as thirty years ago, the world's experts in gastroenterology told us no germs could grow in the acid environment of the stomach. I believe we are still in our infancy in understanding how the biome, interacting with the immune system, diet, and other environmental exposures, is critical in the initiation and propagation of human chronic disease.

I believe this phenomenon to be the root cause of a number of chronic diseases. As a nephrologist, I saw more cases of some chronic diseases in five years than most physicians see in a lifetime, and this unique experience—for more than thirty-five years—helped me piece together connections other more specialized physicians might have missed. I believe the bacteria and yeast growing on the bowels could be the cause of damage to the walls of arteries (atherosclerosis), kidneys (nephritis), skin (psoriasis and eczema), lungs (interstitial pulmonary disease and asthma), nerves (multiple sclerosis, neuropathy of various types), and many others.

The following chapters tackle different sites of these chronic diseases, starting with the lungs.

CHAPTER NINE

CHRONIC DISEASE IN THE LUNGS

One of the best recent publications on the subject of micro-organisms and disease deals with an organ system not yet mentioned in this writing—the pulmonary system. The lungs, like other organs, are vulnerable to a variety of diseases such as infections and malignancies. Diseases that are of unknown cause and specific to lungs, however, may be broadly categorized into chronic obstructive pulmonary disease (COPD), chronic interstitial lung diseases, and asthma and asthmatic bronchitis (or reactive airway disease).

ASTHMA AND BACTERIA

Asthma is a common problem, for both children and older adults, in which there is constriction of smooth muscle in the walls of airways, resulting in poor movement of air in and out of the lungs. The classic physical finding is a musical wheezing noise when a clinician listens to the lungs with a stethoscope.

Asthma can vary from mild to very severe, and it is a major cause of death in the United States. Surprisingly, despite millions of dollars in research by academic institutions and pharmaceutical companies, asthma is still a disease of unknown cause. And because there is no definite cause, there is no definite therapy common to patients with asthma. A group of drugs are used to treat asthma, mostly the same that have been in use since I entered medical practice fifty years ago.

Basically, we give patients steroids to shut off the immune inflammatory response, and we give them drugs that pharmacologically dilate the constricted muscle in the walls of the bronchi in the lungs. For many people, this is sufficient to abort the asthma attack, but often patients develop chronic symptoms and have to return again and again to physicians' offices or hospital emergency departments for breathing treatments consisting of bronchodilator medicines or steroids.

Once in a while, a physician assumes infection might play a part in development of the disease, so antibiotics are given. Some asthmatic patients become chronic respiratory cripples— they cannot eat certain foods or be exposed to certain inhaled substances without developing severe wheezing and shortness of breath. Guidelines are certainly in place for treatment of asthma, but there is no specific way in which all patients are successfully managed.

In 2013, a wise physician from Wisconsin named David Hahn published a wonderful book titled *A Cure for Asthma?: What Your Doctor Isn't Telling You—and Why*. As usual, I did not find the book on a shelf. A patient presented to my office with diffuse joint pain in his hands and feet some months after an episode of bronchitis and pneumonia. He had acquired a copy of Dr. Hahn's book and thought I might like to read it.

Dr. Hahn is an apparently excellent primary care physician

and epidemiologist, who has spent a great deal of time over the past thirty years taking care of asthmatic patients. Much like Dr. Crook learned he could successfully treat a host of disease states by killing yeast, Dr. Hahn learned somewhat by trial and error that he could successfully treat many patients who had severe asthma and asthmatic bronchitis with repetitive courses of azithromycin, a macrolide antibiotic that is an alternative to penicillin.

Dr. Hahn did a very scholarly study of his results in treating asthmatic patients—often severe asthma—with repetitive courses of antibiotics. He specifically used the macrolide antibiotic azithromycin because it is relatively nontoxic and commonly available—but mostly because he saw such startling results with its use. His research and that of others has identified the same chlamydia pneumonia and mycoplasma pneumonia organisms—discussed in the next chapter in relationship to atherosclerosis and vascular disease—to be the likely root cause of the majority of chronic asthma cases. In his experiences as a clinician of nearly forty years, he has found that these bacteria-like organisms are likely the cause of asthma in millions of people around the world. The organisms are responsive to and killed by azithromycin—and likely other antibiotics.

Dr. Hahn has successfully treated hundreds with this therapy, documenting some of these individual cases in his book. Sadly, medical schools and academic institutions have not been able to prove in the laboratory that germs of any specific kind are present in people with asthma and therefore cause asthma. As a result, the recommended therapy for chronic asthma typically does not include an antibiotic.

ASTHMA AND YEAST

My experiences with asthmatic patients differ from those

described in Dr Hahn's excellent book, in that the driving cause for the asthmatic reaction was not bacteria but yeast. Let me share two stories that have stood out in my career, although there are many more such examples.

In an insurance company for which I did consulting, I got to know a nice supervisor pretty well over the months. She was often coughing, but I did not notice until one day when the coughing was especially bothersome, and she looked quite ill. She confessed she had suffered from asthma for several years and that she was now taking five different medicines (inhalers and pills). She thought she might have to give up her job and collect disability benefits fairly shortly.

You know what I was thinking, don't you? I told her about *The Yeast Connection* and the outside possibility that her bowel yeast—not yeast in the lungs—might have something to do with her asthma. She had received over the years numerous courses of antibiotics, along with oral prednisone and other steroids to shut off inflammation, and her asthma had gotten worse instead of better. When I asked, she said she had struggled with vaginal yeast infections from time to time. This of course got my attention.

I told her about Dr. Crook's book and that I would be willing to give her some nystatin if she felt it was worth a try. The truth was that she was so ill she would have tried almost anything to feel better. She read *The Yeast Connection* over that weekend, and came back to work even sicker and more short of breath— but anxious to give the nystatin treatment a try.

I told her—from my reading of Dr. Crook's book—that patients who truly have a large yeast overgrowth in the bowel can sometimes get quite ill when they begin taking nystatin to kill yeast. This was reminiscent of the early days of treating syphilis with penicillin in the 1940s. Many men whose bodies were filled with spirochetes had bad headaches and rashes as the penicillin killed the syphilis organisms. After a few days, symptoms went away, and the penicillin could be continued for as long as necessary to successfully treat the disease. Dr. Crook noted that this same kind of thing can occur when high-volume yeast infestation is treated with nystatin or fluconazole. I told my insurance supervisor she might experience such a reaction if she actually had yeast overgrowth in her bowel.

She began the nystatin on a Friday afternoon. The next day, she had a headache and felt "toxic" and nauseated. I told her it might be the reaction described above and to push on with the nystatin. By Monday afternoon, when I saw her at the insurance office, her headache and toxic feeling were gone. More important, her wheezing and shortness of breath were much less intense. She continued with the nystatin over the next few weeks, and miraculously her asthma symptoms steadily decreased.

By the end of the next month, she had tapered off all five of her asthma medicines, including her steroids, and was free of wheezing. I was amazed, and she was grateful. I think I gave her a short course of fluconazole to consolidate the therapy. She remained free of symptoms as long as she took the nystatin. Her asthma returned on a couple of occasions over the next several years, and each time, her symptoms were relieved by taking nystatin and fluconazole.

My second story has to do with a friend's sister. I had occasion several years ago to care for a dear friend who was dying of cardiomyopathy. Her story alone is most remarkable—because she is no longer dying—but this short narrative is related to her sister, Linda.

Linda was a fairly healthy woman in her fifties who came to Texas to minister to her sister, who was dying of heart disease. We elected to take my friend out of the hospital to die at home, and Linda was assisting with the home management. I made daily visits to the home to listen to my friend's lungs and manipulate the huge bevy of medications she had received in the hospital. My friend administered the power of prayer, and her lungs began to clear after several weeks.

I noticed that Linda coughed incessantly. It was not a loose juicy cough—just a dry irritated cough that seemed to make her uncomfortable but did not slow her down much as she bustled about caring for her very ill older sister. Finally, I asked her about the cough, how long it had been going on, if she had seen a doctor or taken antibiotics, and whether she had gone for a chest X-ray. She assured me she had seen good doctors at her home in Illinois and that her chest X-ray had not shown any cancer or other diseases. She was told she probably had a form of asthma or bronchitis.

I asked how long she had been struggling with the cough, and I was flabbergasted. She had been coughing this way for more than five years. She said it began with a usual cold and that, after the cold, the cough never went away. She had received a couple of courses of antibiotics, which did not take away the cough. She assumed she had asthma and resolved to live with the cough.

I asked if I could listen to her chest with my stethoscope. I heard nothing pathologic. She certainly did not have the wheezing characteristic of asthma, and her lungs seemed perfectly clear. She coughed a half dozen times while I was listening to her chest, making it difficult to listen well, but her pulmonary exam was normal. She had no signs of congestive heart failure, and quite frankly, I had no idea why she had this chronic cough.

The Spirit in the room urged me to tell her about Dr. Crook's book and the outside chance that by killing yeast in her bowel she could possibly stop coughing. I told her about my dialysis patients, as well as the story of my asthmatic friend at the insurance company who had gotten well with nystatin. Linda wanted to try nystatin. She agreed to read *The Yeast Connection*, and I called in her prescription for nystatin.

By day four of the nystatin, Linda's cough ceased. It just stone-cold stopped. When I listened to her lungs, there was a strange quietness in the room. The cough of five years' duration that was refractory to good antibiotics had stopped after four days of a drug that does not get into the blood and could not possibly have arrived in her airways or lungs. I was amazed but not surprised. The interesting thing about Linda is that her cough has never returned. She went home to Illinois as her previously dying sister slowly recovered. If she had been allergic to something in Illinois, it never again caused a reaction.

THE COMMON PATTERN

I hope by now that you see a common pattern in all of this discussion. Bacteria or yeast, through their interaction with the immune system, cause production of products that have a negative effect on human tissues—in this case, the lungs. The result is an often-devastating illness that has no known cause. Since no root cause is identified, the patient is forced to seek therapy for inflammation, which means steroids and many of the drugs used over the past fifty years to treat autoimmune diseases—and to prevent the rejection of transplanted organs.

So how did Dr. Hahn's patients with asthma get better with repetitive use of the antibiotic azithromycin, which kills bacteria? And how did my patient who worked for the insurance company get better with nystatin, an anti-yeast medicine? My answer to this question at this point is that asthma is mediated by the immune system, which makes chemicals that cause the disease. In some cases, the offending organism that initiates the process is a bacterium, and in other cases, the offender may be a yeast. I suspect that both types of organisms can have the same effect on the immune system and cause immune activity to occur. Which organs get damaged by this process is likely a genetic matter, predicted only with a close look at family medical history.

Amazingly, Dr. Hahn has not received recognition for his wonderful work, despite more than thirty years of excellent primary care research in the management of asthma. The reasons for this lack of recognition are numerous, but the most important are related to the fact that those who write guidelines for the care of asthma do not work in the community with boots and gloves in place caring for sick people. I suspect that were Dr. Hahn an academic physician in a medical school he would likely not have written *A Cure for Asthma?*

Academic institutions are strongly influenced by pharmaceutical companies that fund their research. Those who work in medical schools and research centers, writing papers and formulating guidelines, often do not take care of sick people in the community. People like Dr. Hahn, who have spent their careers in the trenches taking care of the very ill, see a different group of patients than do those in medical schools and research centers. The net result of this disparity is that medical truths are often available to those who take care of the sick but are ignored by those who write papers and publish guidelines. It is a sad state of affairs.

I hope those who read this book gain new insights into diseases of unknown cause and recognize that likely hundreds of diseases might be related to immunologic reactions to bacteria, yeast, protozoans, and sometimes viruses.

All the books I have referenced in this writing should serve as a medical library for those who desire to have long-term good health. Tidbits of information in all of them will likely improve the lives of those who incorporate the knowledge in practical ways into their management of health problems. Obviously numerous individuals over the years have come to me with chronic coughs refractory to multiple courses of antibiotics, and have gotten well with nystatin and fluconazole. One of my children has seen a cough of six months' duration go away after several weeks of nystatin. While I still treat bronchitis and some upper respiratory illnesses with antibiotics, like Dr. Hahn has done for treatment of asthma, I almost always give these patients a course of nystatin to take with the antibiotics so they will not be vulnerable to yeast-mediated illness as a consequence.

So, yeast and bacteria affect the lungs, but what about other locations and other diseases? Let's move for a moment to the problem of chronic pain. I'm not going to tell you that all chronic pain can be treated with nystatin. Nevertheless, there is a connection.

CHAPTER TEN

CHRONIC PAIN AND MICROFLORA

annah is a thirty-five-year-old homemaker and mother of two who came to my office at the suggestion of her father, with whom I participated in a Bible study. He told me his daughter was suffering with bad pain in her left leg following an accident several years earlier. She had recovered from the acute injury but developed a relatively rare complication of orthopedic injury called reflex sympathetic dystrophy, or now more commonly known as chronic regional pain syndrome.

The problem typically follows a significant injury to an extremity but can occur in almost any location. What happens is that in the course of an injury, the sympathetic nervous system becomes injured along with the bones and soft tissues, and the patient experiences changes in temperature and color in the injured area as well as rather severe pain. This is an awful problem that creates an almost unparalleled degree of pain. The sympathetic pain may endure for years and has often led to suicide of its victims because of its intensity and duration. It is much like the quality of pain sometimes suffered by patients after an episode of shingles or herpes zoster. Sometimes it is treated successfully with the surgical transection of sympathetic nerves, but even this therapy is often unsuccessful.

When I first saw Hannah, she had suffered left leg pain for nearly five years. Pain and discoloration of her leg ran from her foot to her groin area, and she had associated pain in her vagina and vulva area. She was depressed and miserable, and came to see me with her mother after her father and I had prayed together for her healing.

Hannah was taking near maximal doses of Vicodin and a number of other pain medications of lesser strength. She knew she was hooked on narcotics, but they offered the only relief that allowed her to get through her day. I wanted to be kind, explaining to her and her mother that I was not a pain management physician. I had no magic rabbits up my sleeve.

Still, I was intrigued by a couple of items in her history. First, she had received a course of anti-inflammatory steroids (Medrol Dosepak) once a few years earlier and had actually felt less pain for those couple of weeks. Her physicians, fearing side effects of steroids, would not give her more steroids but continued to give her narcotics. She had received some anesthetic blocks of her left leg nerves, but this therapy was not successful. Also, when she and her family travelled to Colorado and New Mexico for vacation, her pain was significantly reduced. For about ten days on two occasions when living at high altitude, she was able to cut her narcotic dosage in half. That seemed unusual to me, since most pain is aggravated by high altitude and low oxygen concentration.

Quite frankly, I couldn't put that data together with any known cause of her pain. I really didn't know what to do to help. I told her of my experiences with killing yeast in the bowel and remission of various symptoms with nystatin alone. Hannah agreed to read *The Yeast Connection* and do a trial of nystatin.

I gave her a Medrol Dosepak to shut off inflammation and told her she could take two to start if she wanted. I also gave her a prescription for nystatin, not expecting much but hoping for the best. I prayed with Hannah that day and told her that if the Lord wanted her to be well, nothing could stop her from getting better.

I called Hannah after a few days, and she acknowledged that the steroid dose pack gave her some pain relief. I told her she could take a couple of the Medrol Dosepaks but that any good they did would likely be gone within a couple of weeks. What happened, however, is after she took the steroids—while still on nystatin daily—her leg pain progressively diminished. Within a couple more weeks, she had nearly tapered off her Vicodin and was taking much less toxic and safer analgesics.

Amazingly, this was not a short-term effect. Since that time, Hannah continues to do remarkably well. Her pain is minimal now, and her life is much more joyful. The discoloration of her leg has gone, and she has no more vaginal or vulvar pain. I wrote her prescriptions for fluconazole, which also was helpful and allowed her to discontinue nearly all her pain medications.

I was amazed and grateful that God had given this young mother a new lease on life. I'm not sure how it worked, but the patient had a chronic pain syndrome that was in some way made worse by the growth of yeast in her bowel and vagina. Killing her yeast with something as simple as nystatin caused a dramatic improvement.

I'm not saying that killing yeast will make *all* pain go away. My experiences with Hannah and others like her, however, make me wonder if other people who are experiencing chronic pain might be helped with this approach.

Let me tell you about a couple of other patients. Jim is a twenty-something young man who presented to me for evaluation of persistent headaches after a basketball injury. A freshman at a famous university, Jim had been struggling for several months. He had had trauma during the previous year's basketball season and almost immediately thereafter developed persistent headaches. The headaches were bilateral and frontal and occurred almost every day for hours. They were not associated with nausea or unusual visual phenomena, which are symptoms associated with migraines. He had seen several physicians who told him he likely had a concussion.

Six months post injury seemed quite a long time for a teenager to still be experiencing concussion symptoms, but I'm not a neurologist. I had to believe his neurologist was diagnostically correct. The problem was that he was miserable. He was having trouble going to class and making his grades because of the headaches and spaced-out feelings associated with them. He felt he had not been "right in the head," as he put it, for at least six months, and his parents wondered if I could suggest anything that might give him some relief.

I began my discussion by recommending other types of pain medications that might be of value. After examining him thoroughly, I really had no idea why he was having persistent concussion symptoms this long post injury. Lacking any other logical plans, I told him I had seen several patients who had seen some decrease in chronic pain after taking antibiotics and antifungal agents. Jim was anxious to try anything that might be an improvement to all of the therapies he had thus far tried. If his biome (bowel organisms) had anything to do with his head pain, I reasoned that a shotgun approach to treatment would include my prescribing both an antibiotic, like doxycycline, as well as nystatin to cover yeast.

Jim and I prayed for wisdom regarding his illness, and I wrote prescriptions for doxycycline and nystatin, again not very confident that the medicines would do him much good. I prayed and called Jim daily for the next week. He took the medicine faithfully, but a week later he still had close to the same headache pattern.

I felt discouraged but told Jim I would consider changing to another antibiotic. Amazingly, a couple of days later he called to tell me his headaches were gone. After six months of pain, and about ten days of doxycycline and nystatin, a strange illness had run its course.

As a physician, I could only conclude that his biome had changed over the previous ten days to finally remove some toxin or immune system chemical from his bowel, and the headaches ceased. Since that time, Jim has not had a recurrence of his concussion syndrome. He graduated from college and has successfully entered the workforce. I don't know for sure that my medicines contributed to his clinical improvement. I simply know he had a long-term illness that went away when I gave him something that could change his biome and hence his immune responses.

One more story is worthy of mention at this time. Jake, the assistant pastor of a local church, came to me because he had heard I was a physician who did creative things and prayed with patients. His story was similar to Jim's, in that Jake had had chronic facial pain for a couple of years.

Two years earlier, he was riding his bicycle at a pretty fast rate of speed down the access road of a highway. Suddenly, the driver of the car on his left made a quick right turn in front of him. Jake was going too fast to stop and crashed into the automobile's right rear door jamb with his left cheek area. He did not lose consciousness but was badly injured. He likely fractured his left maxillary sinus and had a severe laceration that required some sutures. Thankfully, he did not suffer a closed-head injury and did not develop headaches after the initial pain subsided.

But shortly thereafter, he did develop a chronic severe pain syndrome on the left side of his face. It was similar in intensity to that experienced by Hannah with her leg. He sought help from several neurologists, but MRIs and CT scans of his facial bones did not reveal any obvious reason for his severe pain. He tried all kinds of headache medicines but eventually ended up on Vicodin, which did not control his pain very well.

His neurologists concluded that Jake had a form of trigeminal neuritis as a result of trauma to the soft tissues innervated by the fifth cranial nerve. It was nice to have a definitive diagnosis, but the diagnosis did not cure the pain. He tried a course of medicine that is usually successful in treatment of trigeminal neuralgia, but this also was not successful.

Jake was miserable, and I felt his pain pretty deeply. Obviously, he was a deeply spiritual man and accepted the fact that God was asking him to walk through a deep valley of pain. He had already learned much about suffering and its spiritual value. Nevertheless, he felt the pain robbed him of energy. He would be grateful if anything could help him. I told Jake I had no magic bullets with which to treat him but that I had occasionally seen a patient with chronic pain get better with antibiotics and antifungal medicine. Jake had received one Medrol Dosepak in the two preceding years, but he did not remember if it helped him. He was willing to try a regimen consisting of doxycycline and nystatin preceded by a Medrol Dosepak. He promised to keep a log of his pain pattern.

I was disappointed a week later after the Medrol pack was complete and Jake had no appreciable improvement in his facial pain. He agreed to continue to take the antibiotic and nystatin for a couple more weeks, just to make sure there was no chance of benefit. We had prayed about his pain and asked God to do a miracle, but as usual, I didn't think it likely would see much of an effect.

Quite surprisingly, a couple of weeks later, Jake called to tell me his pain was gone. He wanted to thank me for praying with him and giving him hope. He asked how long he should take the antibiotic and the nystatin. I told him I had no idea how long but that I recommended he continue for at least a couple more weeks. He did so and continued to be pain-free. That was a couple years ago at the time of this writing, and he continues to be healthy, strong, and very physically fit. I have no idea which medication helped him, or if this was simply a great gift from God to one of his servants.

The stories of Hannah, Jim, and Jake gave me confidence that the biome, which extends along the mucous membrane from the sinuses to the anus, might induce biochemical changes that can aggravate chronic pain. Others with pain have responded to a similar therapeutic approach, but the confines of space in this book mean I cannot tell you all of their stories. But Hannah, Jim, and Jake form powerful examples of what can be gained from managing the biome. Not all pain should be expected to remit with such therapy, but the fact that *any* pain syndrome could get better with such an unusual treatment plan is noteworthy.

———

CHAPTER ELEVEN

ATHEROSCLEROTIC VASCULAR DISEASE AND BOWEL MICROFLORA

What about germs and atherosclerotic vascular disease? Heart attacks and strokes get a lot of attention as the most common causes of death from vascular disease. But it is also related to diseases of the arteries of the lower extremities, kidneys, and other organs. For more than fifty years, physicians have written papers suggesting bacteria in the lungs and other organs are possibly responsible for the inflammatory reactions that put into motion damage to the inner linings of the arteries.

Atherosclerosis, which is characterized by thickening of the arteries, is certainly the scourge of our time and likely will be the cause of death for most who read this book. After trillions of dollars of research and thousands of papers on the topic, atherosclerosis is still a disease of unknown cause. We know a lot about who is likely to get the disease, and we are good at pointing out risk factors for atherosclerosis. Nevertheless, when people ask me what causes it, I simply say, "The Nobel Prize has not yet been given for that issue."

I tell my patients the risks for the disease and usually tell them I know of three things that likely are causative for vascular disease: smoke exposure, high blood levels of insulin, and infected teeth and gums. On the surface, none of these has anything to do with the other. They all suggest that some toxin related to these risks is damaging to the intimal lining of an artery.

We think we know that the disease begins with inflammation—a little red streak in the lining of an artery that becomes infiltrated with white blood cells containing cholesterol and other lipids. Over time, the cholesterol from the white blood cells—called macrophages—becomes part of a kind of scab that takes residence in the wall of the artery. We call this scab a plaque, or atheroma. Over time, these scabs become larger in some people and eventually can lead to blockage of blood flow in the area. Much of the testing for vascular disease is designed to tell if there is any decrease in blood flow in vessels that contain these plaques. We routinely do such testing for arteries to the head and legs, and the coronary arteries, in cardiology and vascular surgery offices, as well as during executive assessments as part of corporate wellness programs.

Not known at this time is what makes the lining of the artery get inflamed in the first place. Is it possible gut bacteria and yeast, in influencing the immune system of the bowel, could allow chemicals to be released that damage the lining of arteries? Of course, it is possible, but has anyone proven it? Not as far as I can tell! It is possible that toxins made by bacteria and yeast are absorbed out of the bowel and enter the bloodstream to be distributed widely throughout the body. We know for certain that vascular disease rarely if ever occurs in a ten-year-old, but that certainly is not the case for those over age fifty.

I have been looking at ultrasound studies of the carotid arteries for the past decade or longer, and it is evident there is a specific age when people begin to develop plaque in their arteries. Some individuals do not seem to get this problem, but it clearly is much more common in mature patients than in the young. An aging bowel would certainly be a setup for absorption of toxins that in the younger bowel could not be absorbed. The toxins could come from the organisms or from products made by the immune system in response to the absorbed toxins.

As noted, a number of investigators have concluded over the years that bacteria have something to do with the cause of atherosclerosis. As long as fifty years ago, physicians hypothesized that a small bacteria-like organism called mycoplasma pneumonia (or chlamydia pneumonia) could be the cause of coronary and other vascular disease. Hundreds of medical research papers have been written on the subject, and many researchers today feel that inflammation of the inner lining of arteries has something to do with exposure to this organism.

The reason for this hypothesis is the marked increase in heart attacks and strokes in individuals fairly recently exposed to mycoplasma pneumonia. When people have high antibody titers in their blood to mycoplasma, they appear to be especially vulnerable to rupture of the plaque (scabs) in the walls of their arteries. Something about exposure to the organism results in instability in the lining of an artery, which then becomes vulnerable to the processes that result in a heart attack or stroke.

When pathologists have looked carefully into the composition of the plaque in arteries of patients with heart and vascular disease, they occasionally found evidence of the mycoplasma organisms in the plaque. Most of the time, however, this was not the case. Out of thirty or forty plaques evaluated in one good study in rabbits and humans, there were only a few cases in which the bacteria were discovered in the plaque. The authors were forced to conclude that most arterial plaques have nothing to do with mycoplasma or any other infectious organism.

Based on what is addressed in this writing, however, I would simply say there is no evidence that infection with mycoplasma caused the plaque to form in the first place or to rupture. The many studies mentioned simply showed that in the weeks and months after a mycoplasma pneumonia infection, patients were generally much more likely to have heart attacks and strokes than those who did not have such an infection.

Remember the strep infection in the leg of a rabbit? The strep was in the skin, but the rabbit's kidneys died a quick death because of something made by the rabbit's immune system that secondarily caused the kidney to get sick and die. No strep bacteria were in the rabbit's kidney. There were small immunologic particles that contained an antibody and a tiny dead piece of the strep organisms in the damaged kidneys, but there were no living organisms. Hence, we say that post-streptococcal infection leads to immune damage to the kidney.

If this is true, and mycoplasma pneumonia infection often shortly antedates heart attacks and strokes by a short period of time, it remains possible that immunologic chemicals made at the point of the mycoplasma infection may in fact be the cause of the damage to the lining of arteries. If we doctors can't find evidence of infection, we assume that infection with germs of various kinds is not the cause of the disease. We know, however, that just because no germs are found at the site of a disease does not mean germs have nothing to do with the disease.

How then would one go about trying to find out whether mycoplasma pneumonia via some circuitous immunologic process causes coronary artery disease and stroke? The obvious answer is that we would find out how to suppress growth of mycoplasma with some medication, use the medicine for a number of weeks or months, and see whether heart attacks and strokes diminish over time. Amazingly, despite hundreds of papers dealing with mycoplasma pneumonia and vascular disease, I cannot find one that deals with good therapy of mycoplasma and its effects on vascular disease progression. The reason it hasn't been done, in my opinion, is because we use antibiotics to treat infections. If there is no infection, we assume antibiotics (and antifungal medicines) have no value in treatment.

Is there a good known therapy for treatment of mycoplasma pneumonia? Of course, there is! Hundreds of papers for the past fifty years have demonstrated good effects of at least three classes of commonly used antibiotics in treatment of mycoplasma infection: macrolide antibiotics (erythromycin, azithromycin, clarithromycin), fluoroquinolone antibiotics (ciprofloxacin, levofloxacin), and tetracycline antibiotics (doxycycline, minocycline). All of these offer very effective therapy of mycoplasma, although the macrolides—probably because of overuse in recent years—are recently subject to mycoplasma pneumonia resistance. Mycoplasma is no longer so easily killed by macrolide antibiotics.

Most papers on therapy of mycoplasma pneumonia suggest a two-week course of one of the abovementioned antibiotics. Many articles on the subject, however, discourage using any antibiotic treatment of mycoplasma infections because it is assumed that most people get well from mycoplasma infections with no therapy whatsoever. Of course, most people get well from *any kind of* infection without formal therapy, but that doesn't mean the antibiotic does not change the long-term immunologic outcome of exposure to a germ.

As we know, prolonged use of antibiotics and antifungal agents—not to treat infections in the classical sense of infection—may profoundly affect how the immune system responds to an ongoing exposure to a microorganism. For example, if mycoplasma pneumonia is a chronic contaminant in the airways or some other place in the body, such as the lining of a sinus or the bowel, it could cause ongoing immune activity directed against an important body tissue. This could include the lining of our arteries—a possible explanation for the well-known and written-about relationship that connects mycoplasma pneumonia with atherosclerotic heart disease and stroke.

To address this, experts need to establish and fund a large study in which individuals who have been invaded by mycoplasma—which may include most people who are age seventy or older—be treated for a year or two with tetracycline. The therapy would need to include nystatin to keep yeast from growing during use of the antibiotic. I hope such a study will be set up sometime soon, and perhaps those who read this writing will make it happen. Wouldn't it be wonderful if the prevention of atherosclerosis were to include only an antibiotic, an antifungal agent, and some probiotics? It sounds a lot better to me than angioplasties, stents, and bypass surgeries.

The point is that numerous diseases are likely related to our exposure to the host of microorganisms that line the sinuses, bowels, and airways and interact in critical ways with our very complex immune systems. The reason we don't know this is true—despite the fact that we have had wonderful antibiotics available for nearly a century—is that we use antibiotics only for treatment of infections and not for removal of organisms that stimulate immune damage of the vital organs. Shame on us!

Here I hearken back to the story of rheumatoid arthritis, to explain how this can happen. Remember that in the early days, half of rheumatology professors believed RA was caused by a patient's history of gonorrhea. The other half of the professors didn't think this was right, because they had seen many rheumatoid arthritis patients who never had gonorrhea. The latter group won the argument, so after around 1970, no one even discussed the fact that many individuals had gonorrhea as a predecessor to their cartilage and joint disease.

The end result of fifty years of therapy for rheumatoid arthritis is what we hear every day on our televisions. There are now more drugs than we can name to treat more diseases than we can name with the same style of disclaimers at the ends of the advertisements: "This drug can cause death from cancer, lymphoma, tuberculosis, unusual fungi, and a host of other bad things." Shame on us again! If even some of these conditions can be treated with simple regimens like tetracycline and nystatin, we should identify which patients can be helped—and for how long they might need to take the medicine. Hopefully, help is on the way for the next generation of patients who have diseases of unknown cause.

CHAPTER TWELVE

MALIGNANCIES AND MICROFLORA

ancer is a major cause of death throughout the world. It was the second most common cause of death when I entered medicine in the late 1960s, and it is still the second most common cause of death—behind vascular disease. Malignancies cause untold suffering, and they are incredibly expensive to treat. Billions of dollars have been spent in researching the causes of cancer and finding the best ways to treat it.

After all of this research, while learning much about cancers, we still do not know the immediate triggers that cause a malignancy to develop. For example, we know combustion products are strongly associated with lung cancer development and that alcohol exposure more than doubles the risk of malignancies of almost all internal organs. What we don't know is how these exposures lead to cancer in some people but not in others.

We know that using drugs to suppress the immune system in patients with transplants results in a significantly increased risk of cancer. Could this dysfunction of the immune system be influenced by the yeast and bacteria that grow in the tube? After observing much of what I now know about yeast and its interactions with the immune system, I have often thought of the possibility that activity of microorganisms in the bowel might sometimes be associated with cancer. In this regard, a couple of my patients are worthy of discussion.

Over the years, I have wondered what it is about yeast that allows this type of organism to induce immunologic change that can cause disease in so many different locations of the body. I'm sure Dr. Crook wondered the same thing. Yeasts, it turns out, are very different in appearance than bacteria. Although there is some variation in the physical characteristics of all microorganisms, yeasts are much more structurally complex than the smaller and simpler bacterial cohorts living in our bowels.

Because yeasts have more varying protein markers on their cell surfaces than do bacteria. this appears to cause them to be more likely to influence the host's immune system to make allergic reactions to them. The whole process is probably much more complex than we know, but the fact that books have been written about immune activity related to yeast—and essentially nothing written about immune reactions to bacteria—makes this hypothesis more likely.

After seeing many patients with various conditions, I wondered whether yeast—or other microorganisms—could not only cause distortion of how the immune system works, resulting in unusual disease states, but if yeast could essentially poison the immune system so it could not do its most critical job of protecting from infections and malignancies. In other words, if some chemical made by a yeast or bacteria in the gut were toxic to normal functioning of the immune system, the excess numeric presence of these organisms or increased porosity of the gut could lead to the excess presence of this same chemical in areas where the immune system creates its own biochemical agents—thus compromising the immune system's ability to fight off health dangers like malignancies (cancer).

Let's look at this in more detail. As we know, poisoning of the immune system with immunosuppressant drugs can allow tumors to grow. We have known this for fifty years in the realm of organ transplantation. The drugs that allow us to transplant hearts, livers, lungs, and kidneys all have the disappointing side effect of increasing risk of malignancies. The nightly barrage of pharmaceutical sales advertisements warns us, "This agent can cause lymphoma, cancer, tuberculosis, and other serious illnesses."

The case of the young patient who received a renal transplant from his father—only to learn that a prostate cancer had been transplanted at the same time—bears witness to how suppression of the immune system can lead to malignancy and other illness. The fact that stopping the immune suppressant medicines in that patient led to rejection of the prostate cancer, as well as the patient's kidney, reaffirms this association.

Thus, it's amply proven that drugs like immunosuppressants affect the immune system to such a degree they lead to the abundance of malignancies—largely because the immune system cannot do its job. What if yeast was having the same effect on our immune systems as these immunosuppressant drugs, but we just didn't know it? If bowel yeast can distort the immune system and cause eczema, headaches, fibromyalgia, coughs, and a host of other diseases, can the same yeast sometimes poison the immune system and allow malignancy to develop? A couple of patients and friends are worthy of a brief discussion of this possibility.

LOUISE'S STORY

About twenty years ago, a dear friend, whom I'll call Louise, was found to have ovarian cancer, or mesothelioma, a malignancy of the lining of the intestines and peritoneum. She underwent a total abdominal hysterectomy, but follow-up CT scans revealed the presence of multiple residual tumors. I was busy taking care of kidney dialysis patients, and kidney and heart transplants, but I spent a good deal of time with my friend as she navigated the healthcare system. She prepared for chemotherapy with placement of a port for venous access. I told Louise of my theory that bowel yeast and possibly some bacteria could be at the root of the immune system failure that might have caused her tumor. She agreed to take antibiotics and antifungal drugs along with her initial course of chemotherapy.

The oncology drugs, of course, caused hair loss, nausea, and other symptoms. I trust that they may have suppressed Louise's tumor growth. Her oncologist, however, rightly told her that the chances of a cure for her disease was very small with the drugs he was giving. In the background of this traditional therapy for ovarian cancer, Louise was taking some cephalexin and fluconazole from me. If yeast had anything to do with the failure of her immune system and development of her malignancy, the fluconazole might help restore her immune capacity and perhaps suppress the chance of recurrence of her disease—if the chemotherapy reduced the amount of tumor present.

To everyone's joy, Louise's tumor completely disappeared after her first course of chemotherapy, and she did not proceed with any other oncology drugs thereafter. She continued taking the antibiotics and antifungal agents for a number of months and remained well. Over time, realizing the typical course of ovarian cancer is a recurrence within the first couple of years, she visited her gynecologist and oncologist every few months.

To the amazement of her physicians, she continued month after month to be free of disease. Louise remained disease-free for the next fifteen years and continued to enjoy life, the birth of grandchildren, and great joy in her profession.

Sadly, her disease returned after fifteen years, and she received more chemotherapy. By that time, a number of new anti-cancer drugs were available, and Louise entered into a trial of several. After a few months of receipt of these agents, it was apparent her disease this time was refractory to all chemotherapy. She took some antibiotics and antifungal agents late in the course of the disease, after several courses of chemotherapy, but they were to no avail. Louise went home to be with her Savior more than fifteen years after her disease originally occurred.

Whether the antibiotics and antifungal drugs received twenty years ago influenced her long remission from cancer, we do not know this side of heaven. In the back of my mind has always been the nagging suspicion that her biome had something to do with her disease and the failure of her immune system to reject her malignancy. I have been reluctant to speak of this hypothesis with my physician friends, because it is so far from the mainstream in its philosophy of the cause of disease. The story of one more friend is, however, worthy of adding at this point to the story of cancer and the biome.

JANE'S STORY

Jane has never been my patient but a family friend for years. About a year ago, she developed lower abdominal discomfort and was found to have an ovarian mass. Jane was obviously frightened and surprised but had a hysterectomy and her ovaries removed, along with resection of the mass.

On biopsy, the mass was obviously an ovarian carcinoma. CT scans and MRIs were done to look for evidence of tumors elsewhere. The scan showed some abnormal areas in other parts of her abdomen, and her surgeon examined those areas with an open abdominal procedure. At surgery, her entire peritoneum was studded with small ovarian tumors. She had widespread cancer, and there was no way all of the sites could be removed with surgery. Some of her tumor was removed, but her surgeon explained to Jane and her husband that her only hope of survival was with chemotherapy consisting of several toxic drugs.

I spoke with Jane several times during the course of her illness, praying with her and discussing my ideas that her cancer had grown because her immune system failed to do surveillance. I explained that we don't know what caused her immune system to fail, but we know that for some reason, her immune system stopped recognizing ovarian cancer cells as foreign to her body. When this happened, cancer cells rapidly grew all over her abdomen. I told her about my theory that yeast in the bowel alters immune activity and that it could possibly be a factor in essentially poisoning her immune system. She agreed to a course of nystatin and some fluconazole, while she was beginning her first course of chemotherapy.

I explained that the chemotherapy drugs were relatively toxic and likely decreased the capacity of her immune system to kill her tumor. I did not discourage her from doing the chemotherapy, but she understood that there is a very low total remission rate with use of chemotherapy in treatment of ovarian cancer.

Her intravenous port was placed for IV access, and she proceeded with her first course of drug therapy. At the same time, she began taking nystatin twice per day to kill bowel yeast and fluconazole once daily to kill any other invasive yeast. She had the usual side effects of chemotherapy—hair loss, weakness, and poor appetite. She bravely continued with weekly courses of chemotherapy for the next two months.

A new CT scan was obtained, and to the surprise of her oncologist, the new study revealed a totally clean abdomen. There were not even scars in the areas where tumors were previously located. The best blood test for following patients who have ovarian cancer is measurement of a protein called CA-125. Jane's CA-125 blood test, which reflects tumor volume for ovarian cancer, plummeted from a previous value of 250 down to less than 10 micrograms. She appeared to be free of disease after just one relatively short course of chemotherapy.

No new chemotherapy has been started since that time, which was several years prior to this writing. Jane feels well, and several CT scans done since that time have shown Jane to be free of any disease. Her disease appears to be in remission at the present time. Statistics predict her tumor will be back shortly, but she and I have been praying for a good outcome. It is far too early to tell whether the antifungal medicines or the chemotherapy were responsible for her tumor's disappearance. Only time will tell.

I would like to think her bowel yeast was poisoning her immune system and that, after a few weeks of antifungal therapy, the surveillance abilities of her immune system had markedly improved. Our current plan is to continue her antifungal regimen for one week each month and continue nystatin daily for many months. She will have another MRI of her abdomen in three to four months, and we will know further how her immune system is doing.

Interestingly, she stopped her antifungal regimen for a few weeks after the first normal MRI, and within a couple of weeks had a very symptomatic vaginal fungal infection. It was her first of these for some time, but it reinforced the fact that we all have yeast growing in our bowels and on all of our mucosal surfaces, and that her yeast was growing luxuriantly despite previous antifungal therapy. Wouldn't it be wonderful if we could induce long-term remissions from malignancies with something as simple and inexpensive as antibiotics or antifungal agents? My friend is now about two years post chemotherapy—free of ovarian cancer and its biochemical markers. I will be calling Jane frequently to see how she is doing, and I will continue to pray with and for her.

You might be thinking all of my stories are simply anecdotal and related to luck of the draw. I point out that in almost every case discussed, the symptoms of disease were of long duration and had not responded to various medical regimens in a variety of offices before coming to my attention. In the case of cancer and malignancies, the treatment for microflora was carried out alongside oncology treatments, and bear in mind that the situation was considered hopeless in many of these cases. We cannot, of course, know precisely what instigated remission in these patients—there is so much about the body and our health that we do not know—but I want us to think outside the box about all distortions the biome might cause. Diseases like cancer and atherosclerotic vascular disease are responsible for so many deaths. Is not any potential treatment worth consideration?

As I have stated previously, we allopathic physicians do everything based on scientific method as it relates to the incidence of disease or whether some therapy has a certain effect on a large group of people. If some medicine helps two people out of twenty, but the other eighteen individuals do not respond to the therapy, it is concluded that the therapy is of no benefit. But to that, I say the therapy was of immense value to the two people it helped, and if the therapy was nontoxic and inexpensive, it was worthy of a trial in all twenty individuals. The uniqueness of each of us, and our unique responses to all kinds of medical interventions, should teach us that what works well for one person might not work at all in another. My contention is that if it works at all for anyone, and it is not hurtful or expensive, it is worthy of a try if the patient believes it is worth the try.

CHAPTER THIRTEEN

FINDING THE UNDERLYING CAUSE

B y now, there is ample evidence that yeast and bacteria in the tube can cause ill health—either by evoking an immunological reaction that affects tissue in distant parts of the body (as in the case of Bill's rheumatoid arthritis, chronic pain, and asthma) or by poisoning the immune system and preventing it from doing its job (as with cancer malignancies).

I admit that often I don't know whether bacteria, yeast, or some virus is the culprit for the cascade that ends with immunologic damage to organs and related diseases. When a patient has chronic symptoms of disease and has not been helped by previous therapy, I feel the freedom to initiate a trial of antifungal or antibacterial therapy—and occasionally both—to see whether disease symptoms will moderate.

Over time, patterns have emerged. For instance, I have concluded—perhaps mistakenly—that eczema, chronic coughs, some headaches, fibromyalgia, chronic fatigue, some asthma, and some lupus-like illnesses are in some way related to immune reactions to *yeast*.

On the other hand, rheumatoid arthritis, psoriasis, plantar fasciitis, inflammatory bowel diseases, ankylosing spondylitis, polymyalgia rheumatica, some cases of asthma, and inflammation of the iris of the eye are more likely related to immune reactions to *bacteria*.

Still other diseases don't respond to treatment at all—neither antifungal nor antibacterial therapy. Many patients have not responded to nystatin or antibiotics. I have been especially disappointed with the use of these types of therapy in patients with Parkinson's disease, multiple sclerosis, amyotrophic lateral sclerosis (ALS), and other serious neurologic diseases. I have to conclude that these illnesses do not seem to be related to immune response to yeast or bacteria.

Where do we go from here with this writing? I sincerely hope I do not offend too many colleagues with this document. It is simply my series of observations arising from my care of people very sick with terrible diseases over the past fifty years. I hope that those who read this book will gain new insights into diseases of unknown cause and will recognize that likely hundreds of diseases that are currently of unknown cause will be found to be related to immunologic reactions to bacteria, yeast, protozoans, and sometimes viruses.

One might ask why this is so important. My answer is of course that treatment of disease with antibiotics and antifungal agents is far less expensive and morbid than is treating the same diseases with toxic agents that decrease inflammation. The anti-inflammation drugs may indeed be necessary for a short period of time—like use of Medrol Dosepak and other steroids—but the total cure for diseases of unknown cause likely will be accomplished only with use of antibiotics and antifungal agents that kill the microorganisms that are the underlying cause of disease.

I would like to see hundreds or perhaps thousands of young physicians, who are just beginning the process of seeing sick people and their illnesses, adopt a new kind of thinking as they approach each patient. In my early years in medicine, I spent all of my time learning the names of diseases and how they presented in different patients. When I was seeing patients in those days, I was excited just to be able to name the disease and tell people what the standard therapy would be. It wasn't until I had been a physician for twenty-five years or so that I began to ask myself, "What is the process going on here?" instead of, "What is the name of this disease?" My experiences with Medrol Dosepak, nystatin, and antibiotics only reinforced my new way of thinking.

I am not unique in this thought process. A growing number of physicians practice what is called functional medicine. This discipline has been pushed along by the work of Dr. Leo Galland in New York City and a number of physicians in other parts of the country. Dr. Galland's newest book, *The Allergy Solution*, discusses the role of allergies in the causation of a large number of illnesses. When I read his writings, I am encouraged by my own experiences and the merits of what I have written in this book.

I believe there have always been physicians who think like Dr. Galland, especially those who for years have taken care of sick people. The pressures of the academic health community, fear of criticism, and fear of economic loss often inhibit this type of creative thinking. We clearly need a new kind of thinking in healthcare. Millions of people—especially those who are self-employed or work for companies that do not offer health plans—have no health insurance. Any type of degenerative illness could bankrupt the majority of Americans, who could not easily take on steep hospital or medical bills. It's common knowledge that the current cost of healthcare is far in excess of what the average pocketbook can afford.

We need simple inexpensive treatments of disease. We could centralize payment for healthcare so the government pays for everyone's care. The costs of the system, however, would not go down with such a centralized plan. Costs likely would be even greater—as more people would have the coverage to seek care for complex illnesses. Most drugs cost the consumer and the insurance company several thousand dollars per month. Multiply that cost by each patient's having multiple physicians administering multiple expensive medications, and you have a recipe for financial and medical treatment failure for all.

We must do better. We must find less expensive and less toxic therapies to deal with inflammatory illnesses, and we need to do it in primary care rather than in subspecialty settings. The hypothesis discussed in this writing—that our microflora indirectly causes almost all chronic disease through the activity of the immune system—needs to be explored in the offices of primary care physicians everywhere. Even if a small percentage of patients get totally well with such therapy, this discovery is a wonderful gift. I am blessed to have practiced functional medicine without knowing it had a name. Hopefully many physicians and their patients will have the courage to think creatively when it comes to chronic diseases and discover the benefits of functional medicine. It is time for change.

HAL'S STORY

The story of another interesting patient will perhaps help solidify this type of clinical thinking. About six years prior to this writing, my son, who is a minister, referred to me another young minister of a church in our community. The minister had recently learned he had an incurable liver disease. My son was very concerned for his friend, who had beaten cancer several years earlier but now had a serious liver disease. His physicians told him he would likely require a liver transplant within the next couple of years.

The minister—I'll call him Hal—and his wife agreed to come to my office for a chat, realizing I am certainly not a hepatologist (liver specialist) and that I have no special credentials in gastroenterology. I told my son I would be glad to listen to Hal's story and offer advice in what I call a "ministry visit" at my office.

Hal and his wife came to my office a week later, and their faces were downcast as they relayed the story of his battle with disease over the past few years. After serving a mission in Africa, he was found to have an unusual type of testicular cancer and returned to the United States for therapy. The cancer had metastasized to his lungs and lymph nodes, so he required surgical removal of the testicle and extensive chemotherapy. He did well with this treatment and was declared, after a couple of years, to be free of tumors. On a subsequent lab screening, he was found to have very abnormal liver tests that were previously always normal. It was initially thought he had some type of hepatitis, but his blood tests for hepatitis A, B, and C were all negative. This led to his having a liver biopsy, which unfortunately revealed an inflammatory scarring disease of his bile ducts known as primary biliary cirrhosis (PBC).

Hal and his wife were told quite accurately that PBC is a progressive liver disease of unknown cause in which something destroys the bile ducts throughout the liver, eventually causing the liver to be nonfunctional and scarred. They were told his liver would likely fail over the next couple of years and there was no known therapy to change the course of progression to liver failure and need for a transplant. They were told also that there was no guarantee the disease would not recur in a transplanted liver—because the cause of the disease was not known. The young couple were upbeat and positive because of their faith, but they knew they were in for some difficult times in the next few years.

I told Hal and his wife I had no quick fixes to deal with their problem. But I also shared that I had felt for some time that many liver diseases likely emanated from microorganisms that grow in the bowel—or immune chemicals made in the bowel—as a result of bacterial or fungal processes. I explained how most blood pumped by the heart goes to the head and feet, returns to the heart through large veins, and is pumped again. All blood pumped to the bowel, however, must drain into the liver, where it is processed—and where thousands of proteins and enzymes are made from blood as it slowly passes through the liver.

I told them that if I had primary biliary cirrhosis—or any other diseases of unknown cause invading my liver—I would place myself on an antibiotic like doxycycline and some nystatin to cover yeast. I would do this, hoping that in killing some of the organisms in my biome, I could interfere with whatever was damaging my liver. I told them I would every few months check my liver blood studies as a guide to whether or not my disease was regressing.

Hal and his wife told me they had asked their hepatologist if antibiotics might make his condition better. The physician assured them there were no good studies to show that antibiotics or any kind of chemotherapy had proven useful in preventing the destruction of bile ducts and development of cirrhosis. I asked the young couple to read *The Yeast Connection* so they would have a better understanding of how bowel organisms—or the immune response to bowel organisms—might cause disease in distant organs. They assured me they would do so, and I assumed I would likely not see them again.

Somewhat surprisingly, they called me a week later, telling me they had read *The Yeast Connection* and wondered if I would be willing to prescribe a course of antibiotics as a trial to see if this type of treatment might change Hal's liver enzyme studies. After some soul searching, since I don't usually like to treat patients who are being cared for by other physicians, I agreed to call in to their pharmacy prescriptions for doxycycline and nystatin.

I explained that I liked doxycycline—a tetracycline antibiotic—for bowel organisms because it kills unusual parasites such as malaria and is often used for treating unusual infectious diseases. I also explained that tetracycline antibiotics have been used for years to treat difficult cases of acne and also as an additive to animal feeds to prevent enteric illness in farm animals. I explained that I also don't like to prescribe antibiotics without giving nystatin to prevent growth of yeast in the bowel.

The young couple felt hopeful, and Hal began the doxycycline and nystatin that week. He felt well and tolerated the medicine. I called him every few days to check on him, and he assured me he felt better than he had in a long time. This was encouraging, and I asked him to return to my office in a few weeks to recheck his liver enzymes. To Hal's surprise and mine, the enzyme numbers were much lower and better than they had been several weeks earlier in his specialist's office. It appeared for the first time that Hal's liver cell death was slowing down. God had worked a miracle, perhaps through the effects of the medicines. Hal had no apparent side effects from the medicines, which he continued over the next year as we watched his enzymes return to normal levels.

These events occurred six years prior to this writing. Hal

has continued his work as a pastor and now has a new primary care physician monitoring his progress. He told me recently that he continued taking the medicines for several years and then felt he was likely totally healed from his liver disease and stopped the doxycycline. He has now been off the medicine for more than two years and continues to have normal liver enzyme studies. He has not had another liver biopsy, since there is no indication for this to be done.

Does his apparent response to antibiotics mean all patients with primary biliary cirrhosis could be cured with antibiotics? I doubt it. It does suggest, however, that in selected individuals this simple therapy could help or even lead to remission from illness.

I tell this story only to further encourage those who have incurable processes to maintain hope and to think holistically about what might be going on in their bodies.

TAKING CHARGE OF YOUR HEALTH

We've talked a lot of how the medical community needs to change when it comes to reevaluating the unknown causes of diseases, beginning with out-of-the-box thinking. If you read some of the books I recommend and practice your own out-of-the-box thinking, you can play a role in directing that healthcare. After all, I was introduced to *The Yeast Connection* and *A Cure for Asthma?* because of my patients—and I owe them a debt for it.

You can also take charge of your health more directly. I always tell my patients that all diseases—besides traumatic ones—are caused by too much of something or too little of something. We get sick and die because we are deficient in some key substance or because we are exposed to excess amounts of something else—or both simultaneously.

This sounds simplistic—and it is—but I have trouble thinking of any common diseases that don't fit into the above categories. We need to ingest all kinds of nutrients—including vitamins, minerals, proteins, fats, and carbs—as well as hundreds of proteins, enzymes, and hormones that are made in the body and are necessary for life. Cortisol, thyroid hormone, and a host of other hormones are a testimony to this fact. When we do proper health screening, we usually measure only a tiny fraction of all key nutrients, hormones, and enzymes that are necessary for life.

So, any patient who comes to my office with symptoms of some disease could be viewed as someone whose body is missing something that needs to be replaced. Some deficiencies are more common than others, and to gauge those, we typically order blood, urine, or other body fluid analysis—thyroid hormone, for instance. But there are thousands of nutrients we don't measure routinely and thousands of others that don't even have names—deficiencies of any of these, or combinations of deficiencies, could cause diseases.

On the other side of the scale is the issue of things that poison us. This could include too many of the nutrients mentioned above or too much of anything that poisons the human system and causes ill health. This includes all infections, as well as excess production of hormones, such as thyroid hormone, adrenal hormone, or parathyroid hormone. This category can include lipids such as cholesterol, which we treat as a metabolic poison and use drugs like statins to reduce its production in the liver. This group can also include things we breathe, such as pollution or cigarette smoke, and what we drink, like plastic contaminant particles in water. It also includes foods of all kinds that can cause sickness through toxic or allergic reactions, like my patient with tomato sensitivity.

Not all of these poisons or deficiencies are out of your control. In the 1980s, when I shifted from taking care of the sick and dying to becoming a community lecturer in health and wellness, I began asking this: "Are there behavioral overtones to this patient's symptoms?" In other words, was this patient doing (or not doing) something that was causing the pathology I was seeing?

In Part 3, let's take a look at behavioral patterns that influence health, and how you can take care of your body and its various microflora—starting now.

PART THREE

CHAPTER FOURTEEN

BEHAVIORS THAT INFLUENCE HEALTH

esides killing germs and manipulating the immune system with drugs, are there behavioral issues that influence health? Yes, of course there are. By this time in human progress, most of us know that if we overeat, smoke, drink too much whiskey, or drive without seatbelts, we can expect to have a shortened life span. We all know genetics are important, and likely—from data derived from identical twin studies—influence nearly 75 percent of health outcomes. Nevertheless, even influencing outcomes by 25 percent, human behavior is hugely important in its influence on health and longevity.

With the cost of healthcare rising annually, we cannot allow ourselves to ignore health-related behaviors. It occurred to me as early as the 1980s that we simply could not afford to allow vital organs to die and then replace them with transplants. I recognized that the vast majority of my kidney dialysis patients had no business being in kidney failure and on dialysis. Almost all had long suffered from Type 2 diabetes before I met them.

Most were thirty pounds to one hundred pounds overweight for most of their adult lives, and this led to diabetes. About 5 percent of people with Type 2 diabetes will ultimately develop kidney failure and need dialysis or a transplant. Abnormal body composition—too much stored fat—was the ultimate cause of failure of these patients' kidneys.

By the mid-1980s, I was convinced we must do a better job of managing body composition—particularly excess fat storage—if we were to reduce healthcare costs. I knew intuitively that many other diseases besides kidney failure were related to excess fat storage. The list is almost endless but includes orthopedic illness, hypertension, most malignancies, obstructive sleep apnea (which causes its own set of related disease problems), Type 2 diabetes, hypogonadism, menstrual abnormalities, digestive disorders, and a host of lesser problems. Clearly, as I deduced back in 1985, if we can't manage body composition, we can't manage health—or the costs of healthcare.

I began a journey that has lasted for many years and to some extent continues at the time of this writing. As a nephrologist, who used dialysis machines to typically remove ten to fifteen pounds of fluid, three times per week, from patients with kidney failure, I knew scale weight was not a very good measure of excess body fat. We needed better tools than bathroom scales to tell us how much body weight was fat and how much of it was lean.

I took a broad interest in various types of equipment designed to measure body composition rather than body weight. These included a Whitmore Volumeter (for underwater weighing), bio-impedance equipment (devices that predict body fat content by passing a low-voltage current through the body), ultrasound units, skin calipers of various types, and finally DEXA scanners, which use low-dose radiation (X-rays) to measure body fat, bone, and muscle content. The latter meets the standard of excellence for measurement of body composition.

I unexpectedly found myself employed as the director of a busy obesity treatment and weight loss program that would ultimately serve more than 30,000 patients over the years. My partners and I recognized that almost all of our chronic kidney failure patients had kidney failure because of diabetes. Most of these patients had developed diabetes because of being obese or substantially overweight for long periods of time. It was only natural for us to be interested in formal programs that taught patients how to successfully manage body weight and hopefully avoid becoming diabetic.

Our program was very scientifically based, and included both specific diets and behavioral programs. While continuing to work as a nephrologist, I became a lecturer and writer on the subject, teaching classes four nights a week for several years—always working to influence change in human behavior in ways that led to decreased fat storage and improvement in body composition. Here I summarize what I have learned about health and fitness into what I call the three great truths.

MANAGING BODY COMPOSITION

The first great truth of health and fitness is that it is absolutely vital to manage your body composition—the amount of muscle, fat, and bone.

I wish I could tell you my Obesity and Risk Factor Reduction Program was a blazing success. It certainly was not. It helped lots of people, for sure, but the vast majority lost fifty pounds and regained sixty. I learned that management of body composition made management of kidney failure and kidney and heart transplants seem like child's play. Without dragging out the explanation, I concluded—after many years of making videotapes, writing textbooks, formulating food laboratories, giving lectures, and seeing patients in outpatient clinics—that the management of obesity is certainly not a diet program.

Obesity is first of all strongly influenced by genetics—at least 75 percent of the problem. Those who have overweight parents are much more likely to also be overweight. Composition management, however, needs to be thought of as an integration of three distinct but interrelated components: 1) education, 2) accountability, and 3) wise use of tools related to education and accountability.

EDUCATION

I've learned that if patients are not educated on the issues surrounding body composition, they have little chance of a good composition after finishing a diet program. They might lose weight on the program, but after a time can return to a weight even greater than at the start of the program. For weight loss to stick, people have to understand that the changes in activity, record keeping, and nutrition need to be lifelong.

They also need to understand that weight loss is not necessarily fat loss. Weight loss can consist of some fat loss, but most of the time, when people lose weight, they also lose bone and muscle along with fat. Loss of bone and muscle is not a good goal for anyone. (Dialysis patients often lose twenty pounds of fluid without losing one ounce of fat.) Conversely, I have seen people gain fifteen pounds of lean mass—bone and muscle—without gaining one pound of fat. With better understanding of healthy management of these different tissues, more patients achieve and maintain weight-loss goals.

ACCOUNTABILITY

People in weight-loss programs also have to be accountable to someone or some system—often for the rest of their lives—if they hope to have a permanent change in composition. This is the reason all great weight-loss programs incorporate a maintenance plan. People are more likely to change, and maintain that change, in all sorts of human endeavors when accountable for their behaviors—not just to themselves but to others around them. This is a fundamental fact of human life. In the Christian Bible, the apostle Paul, in the Book of Romans, bemoans that he did what he *didn't* want to do, and didn't do what he *did* want to do—and that he needed a lot of help to live the right way most of the time. The Roman Catholic Church learned centuries ago that those who come to confession on Fridays are much more likely to live in discipline than are those who aren't so accountable.

Telling someone or some system what we did and did not do is important if we are going to be successful. All of our successful weight-loss patients entered maintenance plans in which they recorded energy balance in their notebooks, and checked in with nursing staff on a regular schedule. A great weight-loss program always employs a good long-term accountability feature to encourage patients and remind them of the tools of success for maintaining healthy composition.

TOOLS FOR EDUCATION AND ACCOUNTABILITY

Finally, we involved in the management of body composition learned that good tools needed to be made available as an outgrowth of education and accountability—that is, if patients were going to change and stay changed. This included record-keeping forms, athletic equipment, diet supplements, unique food products, fitness center memberships, and a host of other ancillary items to influence patients to apply what they learned and agree to be accountable for their accomplishments.

I learned over the years that losing body fat, and maintaining muscle mass and bone mass, is a terrific challenge and that many people have a tough time doing it. I notice that young people today seem to work much more diligently than those of my generation to stay fit and maintain good body composition. It remains to be seen whether or not this young, fit generation will do as well as they pass into middle age and older years.

Having experience of more than forty years with high-quality weight-loss programs, I am convinced that good body composition is critical to the health of almost every individual—and that body composition management is one of the greatest challenges in American medicine. There is so much to learn to be a good manager of one's body composition. The basic equation for management of body composition consists of the following:

To lose fat without wasting muscle and bone, one must raise dietary protein intake while restricting calories of energy coming from fats, carbohydrates, and alcohol. At the same time, one must increase an expenditure of energy through various types of physical activity to create deficits in energy. The deficits result in excess utilization of body fat and, thus, the desired result.

This might sound like exercising more and eating less, but it is more complex. What one eats more of and what one eats less of are critically important to healthfully lose fat without wasting tissues that are important to good health. Only a quality education coupled with a good accountability program and wise use of tools allow accomplishment of safe reduction in body fat stores.

YOU ARE WHAT YOU EAT

The second great truth related to health and wellness is that, to a large extent, you are what you eat. I learned in the early 1980s that I had escaped medical school and years of residency without knowing very much about food composition. It was painfully evident, as I became a lecturer for a weight-loss program, that I had better learn a lot about nutrition or I would not be teaching anybody anything for very long.

I learned that not only the overweight need to understand food and its composition. All of us need to know more about what we eat. For many years, I asked all of my executive exam patients to complete a food frequency questionnaire as part of their annual examination. My patients and I learned quite a lot from this. Too many patients learned from completing this tool that more than 20 percent of their weekly calories came from ethyl alcohol. Most patients were eating far too much fat and simple carbohydrates with too little protein. Over time, we learned that this type of diet causes elevations of blood insulin levels and creates the nutritional background for Type 2 diabetes.

Like most things in life, "if you can't measure it, you can't manage it." I found that knowing what my patients and I consume was a big deal, and it made me a much more complete physician and educator. The big problem with nutritional teaching is that there are so many educational inputs from multiple sources—from government agencies to *Ladies' Home Journal* to television news programs. It became apparent that most issued similar messages about nutrition, but that none knew for sure exactly what each of us should be eating.

This is because nutrition studies were not comprehensive, but also because individuals have unique nutritional needs. Nutrition programs, some sponsored by government agencies and others by commercial weight-loss programs, have little scientific evidence for widespread success of any specific diet regimen. What has been recommended at high levels has often changed 180 degrees over time. It is astute to recognize that what is good for one person is not necessarily good for another. This is especially true for calorie intake between individuals of the same size. Caloric needs can differ by more than 1,000 calories per day in three different people of the same muscle and bone mass.

Over time, I viewed all foods as containing combinations of the four basic nutrients: fats, carbs, proteins, and alcohol. I needed to learn the general amount of each of these in the various foods I was consuming. It is amazing how few people know for sure what is in their food and how it might affect their fat storage or overall health. Obviously, thousands of books have been written on the subject, but most of the time, only dieticians and college students studying nutrition have the foggiest idea what is in their food.

Our recommended nutrition program for patients in our clinic was in line with the advice in four important books on the subject of weight loss: These include *Dr. Atkins' Diet Revolution*, *The Zone Diet*, *Sugar Busters!*, and *The South Beach Diet*. These books share that, to lose weight and have good nutrition, one needs to increase dietary protein while decreasing calories from carbohydrates, fats, and alcohol. It is much simpler to be healthy when we understand what is in food and quantitatively how much is going down our tubes in a given period of time. I'm better at monitoring my food intake now than I was forty years ago, but I still have a lot to learn.

If the big four—carbohydrates, fats, proteins, and alcohol—are challenging to learn, think how hard it is to gain knowledge about vitamins, trace minerals, and thousands of other "micro-stuff" in foods. Since these are of importance in health maintenance, we need to know about them as well. By the early 1990s, I finally had to sit down and write a textbook on the subject for my obesity clinic patients. *Knowing Your Body Weight*, about basic nutrition, is available through my office to patients who are in an active weight-loss program.

The basic premise of that text is that our bodies are energy-demanding machines. We must eat to supply energy to the system, and also to provide nutrients that repair and replace what is damaged and injured over time. Both processes are important. The concept of energy balance is simple, but learning what influences energy balance requires work on the part of each individual. Very few Americans are adept at keeping an energy balance record as a part of their management of body fat. Even fewer understand the various components of energy output or energy input, and how we can manipulate those to better manage our fat stores.

Central to any discussion of energy balance is an understanding of food composition as well as the energy values of the various components. We now have excellent food frequency software programs that can be our teachers in this regard. I hope that all who read this will avail themselves of an opportunity to complete the clinical NutraScreen product of a company called Viocare—an online dietary questionnaire about food frequency. It costs only a few dollars to do the screening, and you will be surprised at what you can learn in less than thirty minutes of data entry.

PHYSICAL FITNESS

The third major division of the health-and-wellness equation is physical fitness.

Prior to the mid-1980s, little was written about physical activity and health. Since then, a host of studies have been published on this subject. In 1987 in the *New England Journal of Medicine*, Dr. Ralph Paffenbarger published a study that forever changed the way we feel about exercise and its effect on longevity. He and his colleagues looked at more than 17,000 male Harvard University alumni of a broad range of ages. They sent out questionnaires to all of these gentlemen, asking them about the following: 1) how many miles they walked in a week, 2) how many stairs they climbed in a week, 3) how many hours of light sports (like doubles tennis) they played in a week, 4) how many hours of heavy sports (like full court basketball) they played in a week, and 5) how much they weighed. With this data, researchers could calculate how many calories of energy these gentlemen burned during various types of activities.

Over the course of more than twenty years, researchers accumulated data on death rates from heart disease, cancer, and accidents in these subjects. The results were most interesting. During the twenty-plus years, about 1,600 of the men died of various diseases (about 8 percent death rate). The data showed a linear decrease in death rate for each calorie of energy expended by these men through about 2,000 calories of expended energy per week—the equivalent of walking about fifteen miles per week for most of them. At a level of more than 2,000 calories per week of expended energy, physical activity had a continued benefit on longevity up through about 3,500 calories per week of exercise. With more than 3,500 calories per week of expended energy, death rates in that study increased slightly.

Therefore, some exercise is very beneficial, but above a certain level of energy expenditure, exercise can actually be harmful. Interestingly, there was not much difference in death rate for different types of exercise. Walking twenty miles per week had just a slightly less beneficial effect on death rate than did playing full court basketball for several hours per week. The data were quite clear, and subsequent studies have shown the same results. Up to a point, a good way to live longer and better is to be physically active. It doesn't make too much difference what type of exercise you do. As long as the activity doesn't hurt you in some way, it likely enhances your ability to live long and well. It is certainly possible to do too much activity and sustain stress-related damage to tissues. Sadly, many individuals don't come close to expending even the first 2,000 calories per week.

Other investigators have expanded on this basic knowledge. Drs. Kenneth Cooper and Stephen Blair, in the late 1990s, published another most interesting paper on a related subject. They looked into the issue of capacity to do work versus longevity in healthy adults. They followed about 10,000 men and 3,000 women for nearly fifteen years, looking at their capacity to do treadmill exercise (a standard time test). They looked at death rates from heart disease, cancer, and accidents in this group of people.

As you might expect, the very fit people outlived the very unfit people. Perhaps unexpected is that the men who were able to complete only six minutes on a treadmill test had a death rate nearly four times that of men able to complete fourteen minutes of the same protocol. For women, the data were even more dramatic. The women who could complete only six minutes on the treadmill protocol had almost five times the death rate of women who completed fourteen minutes. Fit people outlive those who are unfit, and the relationship is pretty linear.

These two studies changed the way I taught fitness and health to my patients. My theological take on the data is that

God intends us to move about in our daily lives and not sit all day in offices. Up to a point, the more we move, the longer we get to live. The data from Drs. Cooper and Blair suggests we should do some of our activity in ways that make us get hot and sweat a little—riding bicycles, jogging, playing sports, or other high-intensity activities. Most important, however, is simply seeking to be physically active.

POISON PREVENTION

Good body composition, good nutrition, and good fitness—what else is important to good health? Sadly, as I learned many years ago, one can be very fit and lean, and have perfect nutrition, and still end up getting very ill and even dying at a young age. The reason for early death in an otherwise healthy young person is almost always some kind of poisoning.

Let me explain. As noted previously, all disease is finally related to too much or too little of something. Too little of something could be a nutrient deficiency or an important hormone not being produced. Too much could mean too much nutrition, too many hormones or chemicals—like the immune system chemicals—or too much of a variety of microorganisms like bacteria, yeast, viruses, or protozoans. Most of this book is a discussion of internal poisoning caused by the immune system as it responds to the ultimate cause of poisoning—germs. So, preventing poisoning is key to good health.

Some poisons are environmental chemicals to which we are exposed, like household cleansers, herbicides, insecticides, solvents, and combustion products. Even minimal exposure to some can take a toll on health. Many medically necessary nutrients and vitamins can be toxic to the body. This is especially true for fat-soluble vitamins like Vitamins A, D, E, and K. Minerals like iron are necessary for production of hemoglobin and for health of other enzyme systems. Excessive iron, however, can build up in tissues and cause heart failure, liver failure, or pancreatic failure with diabetes. Clearly, too much of a good thing can be very bad. Other toxins are generated in the body, like various hormones and enzymes sometimes produced in excess. And too much cortisol can have a negative effect on the system. Excessive production of thyroid hormone, adrenal gland hormones, parathyroid hormone, testosterone, and many lesser-known substances can make a person very ill.

Cholesterol is a classic example of an internally generated substance that can end up in undesirable places. Cholesterol is produced in the liver as it receives orders from other parts of the body that more is needed. I personally don't consider cholesterol a toxin, but very high levels of this substance are associated with atherosclerotic vascular disease and other health problems.

The point of all of this is that despite perfect body composition, nutrition, and fitness, people can get very sick and die because of diverse kinds of poisoning or toxicity. Thousands of books have been written on this subject, and poisoning often sends people to doctors' offices.

Good health screening, which my partners and I have been blessed for many years to provide, is mostly about looking for evidence of toxicity that may be compromising a patient's health. This includes blood levels of iron, lipids—like cholesterol, insulin, lipopolysaccharide, sugar, thyroid hormones, female and male hormone levels—and a host of other chemicals. All of these should be measured as frequently as a patient's physician feels measurement is needed to help the individual maintain optimal health.

Much of the responsibility for avoidance of toxins resides

with the individual, particularly when it comes to what one puts into the body because of addiction or for stress relief. The biggies in this category are well known to us. My top four in this category are smoke and combustion products, ethyl alcohol, addictive drugs like heroin and cocaine, and prescription medications of all kinds.

Most of us have been around long enough to know combustion products grossly shorten life. We smoke to inhale nicotine or marijuana, but it is the smoke products' tars and other stuff that damages body tissues. Most smokers think lung damage is the main disease related to smoke exposure. The lungs are at the front door of smoke damage, but the majority of damage is done to internal organs like the urinary bladder and thousands of miles of artery linings that connect everything together. Not one single tissue in the body is not damaged by smoke products. Nearly every organ in the body, including kidneys, heart, liver, pancreas, uterus, and prostate glands, is negatively affected by chronic smoke exposure. Firemen have a higher mortality than policemen for a good reason—toxic exposure to chemicals and smoke.

Nicotine is not much of a toxin, although it can raise blood pressure somewhat. I have always taught that it is not dumb to use nicotine, but it is dumb to breathe smoke to get the nicotine. We have to find better ways to use nicotine. Most efforts to provide smokeless nicotine have resulted in problems even worse than those acquired from chronic smoke exposure. Vaping is the recent scourge of our young people, and it has caused the deaths of thousands. Nicorette gum has been the mainstay of stop-smoking programs for many years, offering the safest way for smokers to grossly reduce their smoke exposure while slowly tapering away their need for nicotine.

Various kinds of alcohols, such as methanol, are quite toxic, but ethyl alcohol has occupied a privileged position for thousands of years. It is toxic, but its toxicity is harder to measure over a short period of time. Its main societal problems are related to drunkenness and its effects on motor vehicle accident deaths, troubled marriages, and decreases in workplace productivity. Its medical effects are huge but mostly ignored by the public, which has had a love affair with the social benefits of ethanol for centuries.

Almost all malignancies known to mankind are more than doubled in frequency in those who drink ethanol daily. Breast cancer is almost three times more prevalent in women who drink a couple of alcoholic drinks per day than those who do not. Some potential health benefits come from moderate alcohol exposure, but they are meager compared to the toxicity—and loss of organ function and life—related to excessive alcohol exposure.

The problem with the phrase "excessive alcohol exposure" is that when we begin drinking at a young age, we have no idea what might be considered excessive. We don't know who is likely to become an alcoholic and who is not—except perhaps through genetic history in which there are many alcoholics in the family and therefore a marked increase of risk for the disease in those who choose to drink alcohol. Most family members are aware of the familial risk, but drinking often begins anyway. Even the definition of "alcoholic" is often confusing, generally accepted as being one who engages in chronic use of alcohol despite negative health or sociologic consequences.

For years I have said we need sedative-hypnotic drugs that are less toxic and addicting than ethyl alcohol. Unfortunately, sedative-hypnotic pills of various kinds (Valium, Xanax, Librium, and so on) have drawbacks, and are not a much better alternative for the societal costs and medical toxicity of ethanol.

While good body composition, good physical fitness, and good personal nutrition are critical to good health, they can all be trumped at anytime by toxic exposures. As I have often said in lectures to various groups, "You can have perfect body composition, perfect nutrition, and perfect fitness, but if your wife slips a little arsenic into your morning cup of coffee for a few months, you can expect a bad ending—despite your being in excellent health." In the final analysis, the main reason we need physicians and nurses is to deal with the identification of and complications of various toxicities. I guess this means I will always have a job.

In the next chapter, let's look at a few more issues that impact long-term health. These are not as specific as diet and exercise, and indeed are often ignored by those looking to get into good physical shape, but they play starring roles in overall happiness.

CHAPTER FIFTEEN

ISSUES THAT IMPACT LONG-TERM HEALTH

While body composition, nutrition, physical activity, and avoidance of toxins are all important in regard to health maintenance, other issues that influence long-term physical health include quality and quantity of sleep as well as spiritual well-being. These areas of focus are of equal or even more importance than the physical aspects of staying healthy.

Maintenance of good quality and quantity of sleep, as well as nurturing of spiritual awareness, are of supreme importance—but often overlooked and worthy of discussion here. If everything from a health perspective is done diligently by an individual but there is little attention to spiritual wellness and sleep quality, the result could be poor overall health.

SLEEP

Sleep, obviously, is a necessity for all people. My life has been marked since undergraduate days by short nights and long days.

I guess that, while I knew sleep to be necessary, I was never taught its importance to the maintenance of good health.

During the past thirty years, a great deal of beneficial research has been done in understanding the importance of sleep to health maintenance. There is little doubt that quantity and quality of sleep are both critical to good health. The health of the cardiovascular and immune system is strongly influenced by sleep patterns, and mental health deteriorates rapidly with sleep deprivation. Since almost all of us will die of some dysfunction of the cardiovascular system or immune system, and sleep deprivation results in dysfunction of these systems, it follows that poor quality or quantity of sleep is very costly.

Add to this factor the number of sleep-related deaths from auto accidents and household incidents, and you reach a relatively huge number of deaths influenced in some way by disordered sleep. Motor vehicle accidents very often occur with individuals who are sleep-deprived and doze off at the wheel. Most people know this, but we rarely talk about it. As they say, life goes on, whether you had a good night's sleep or not. I wonder how many countless people right now are driving around the highways and byways having had little or no sleep the night before. It's scary!

Quality of sleep is nearly as important as quantity of sleep. We know this because of the large number of scientific sleep studies over the past half century. With good sleep laboratories, it has been possible to thoroughly evaluate human beings and animals as they sleep. Different stages of sleep have been identified, and each stage is important in health maintenance.

Perhaps the best way to look at disordered sleep is to notice what happens physiologically and biochemically as a result. One great cause of illness is obstructive sleep apnea. A person with this disorder experiences partial or total blockage of the upper airway during inspiration while sleeping. The blockage is usually caused by a too-large tongue, which is a common complication of obesity.

With sleep apnea, the tongue falls into the throat and impedes normal breathing. When the obstruction occurs, the autonomic nervous system kicks in to make the patient wake up and breathe. This phenomenon can occur a few or many times per hour, resulting in an inadequate sleep experience. A patient may be in bed for eight hours but in fact get only two hours of sleep.

Lack of sleep can result in high blood pressure, cardiac arrhythmias, clinical depression, diabetes, and all kinds of immune system dysfunction, and secondarily can cause poor work performance and strained interpersonal relationships. I have seen hundreds of patients reverse high blood pressure with effective treatment for obstructive sleep apnea. It's hard not to wonder how many sudden nocturnal deaths might be caused by cardiac arrhythmias precipitated by upper airway obstruction.

Numerous medical studies have documented immuno-logic dysfunction related to poor quality or quantity of sleep. If immune dysfunction causes cancer, then obstructive sleep apnea and related disorders are likely responsible for a great deal of malignancy that plagues the population. Obstructive sleep apnea can be caused by various problems other than obesity. Recurrent nasal obstruction from nasal trauma, nasal allergies, chronic sinus infections with drainage, or hypertrophy of turbinate bones in the nasal cavity can all cause obstructed breathing patterns during sleep.

Treatment of obstructive sleep apnea has become a major area of effective research. The gold standard at the present time is a breathing device that opens the upper airway by forcing air down the windpipe (trachea) during sleep. The procedure is called continuous positive air pressure (CPAP). With CPAP, the obstructed patient's every effort at inspiration results in the breathing machine forcing air under pressure into the back of the throat and down the windpipe. CPAP overcomes the blockage—caused by a large tongue or blocked-up nasal passages—allowing the patient to receive air (oxygen) under pressure into the depths of the lungs.

CPAP equipment is activated by every breathing effort of the patient and results in wonderfully restful sleep—as long as the patient can tolerate the machine's mask and its feeling of pressure. I have known hundreds of patients who were experiencing unrestful sleep due to obstruction but had a marked improvement in overall health after using CPAP. Not everyone who has sleep apnea or sleep-disordered breathing requires CPAP, but it has been lifesaving for many.

A second potential treatment for obstructive sleep apnea is a small mouth appliance placed in the mandible during sleep. The appliance allows the tongue to be moved forward in the mouth and away from the back of the pharynx. This is a bit uncomfortable for some people, but it allows the airway to remain open and results in restful sleep, lowered blood pressure, and fewer heart rhythm problems. For those who cannot tolerate the CPAP mask or wear an oral appliance, a number of surgical procedures have corrected severe disordered sleep.

Surgery to reduce the volume of the tongue has become very common as a treatment of airway obstruction. It is obviously painful, and most people would rather try anything rather than go to surgery for a sleep problem. Nevertheless, removal of obstruction in the nose, posterior soft palate, uvula, or tongue can be lifesaving and result in wonderful sleep quality.

Most people with obstructive sleep apnea are identified by

their spouse or bed partner—or when others who observe that they have stopped breathing while asleep. Snoring is a part of sleep apnea, but the vast majority of patients who snore do not have obstructive sleep apnea. Almost everyone who has sleep apnea snores, but the opposite is not true. Suffice it to say that a good night's sleep is a major component of the behavioral management of health.

A number of good books discuss the importance of sleep and how to maintain good sleep hygiene.[7] All large cities now have specialists in sleep medicine, and almost all of them have informative pamphlets and handouts that teach the public how to get restful sleep. For anyone suffering from obstructive sleep apnea or getting poor quality sleep, a visit to a sleep specialist may prove very valuable.

MINDFULNESS OR SPIRITUAL HEALTH

Along with good sleep in the quest for optimal health is an area referred to as mindfulness, or state of mind. As a Christian, I usually refer to this as spiritual health.

What the heck is spiritual health, and is there any scientific evidence that shows matters of the mind influence health outcomes? There is much evidence that state of mind and related responses to stress strongly influence the immune system and overall health. Studies done long ago on rats and rabbits showed conclusively that animals placed in stressful situations—in which they could not change the stress or change their environment—did poorly from an overall health stand-

---

7   Some well-written books on the subject include *The Sleep Solution: Why Your Sleep Is Broken and How to Fix It* by Dr. W. Chris Winter and *Why We Sleep: Unlocking the Power of Sleep and Dreams* by Matthew Walker.

point. Tumors grew better in stressed rats than in rats that had better environmental control.

You might wonder what mechanism is at work that allows good spiritual health to influence health outcomes? Most experts in this area believe a number of human hormonal systems are activated during life's stresses. The biggies in this regard are adrenaline and other catecholamines, cortisol and all steroids, dopamine and other pressor substances, and glucagon and other agents that raise blood sugar levels. All of these are God-given chemicals designed to save us in stressful situations. All, in my opinion, were designed to be released into our blood transiently—with a rapid return to basal levels. None was intended to be produced chronically in high amounts.

The potential results of too much adrenaline and sympathetic nervous system activity are high blood pressure, skipped heartbeats, and abdominal and bowel problems. The results of too much cortisol and other steroids can include weight gain, high blood pressure, diabetes, acneiform rash, osteoporosis and other bone disease, cataracts and other eye diseases, and immune system suppression. Excess dopamine can cause hypertension and cardiovascular rhythm disturbance. Too much glucagon can result in diabetes. There is likely no end to the list of what can happen in a stressful situation from which there is no easy escape.

What can we do to best manage chronic unresolved stress? Opinions differ, but excellence in all of the areas discussed earlier in this chapter will help us greatly in our battle with stress—leanness, athleticism, nutritional excellence, and avoidance of environmental toxins can all go a long way in helping people manage stresses.

While all of these factors are important, none is as useful, in my opinion, as having an intimate relationship with the God of the universe. Prayer has been shown in large studies to positively affect outcomes of various diseases and recovery rates following surgical procedures. For me as a Christian, intimacy with God through Christ is my best medicine at all times. You might conclude that this is some kind of hokey crutch to help me get through tough times. The truth is that I can do all things through Christ who strengthens me, and I make it a habit to pray without ceasing at every opportunity.

A number of other Christian and Jewish scriptures, as I abide in them and allow them to influence my spirit, have helped me through life's storms. Psalm 23 is famous in this regard, and Psalms 27, 18, and 1 are all examples of stress-relieving scripture. I have made it a habit to memorize scripture throughout my advanced years, and this endeavor has blessed me immeasurably. I commend it to you wholeheartedly as a great reliever of stress. I have little doubt that all the hormonal systems are positively affected by prayer and scripture memory.

Three or four scriptures have been especially meaningful for me over the years. The first is from the little letter to the Philippians in the Christian New Testament.

Be anxious for nothing, but in everything by prayer and supplication, with thanksgiving, let your requests be made known to God; and the peace of God, which passes all understanding, will guard your hearts and minds through Jesus Christ. (Philippians 4:6 NKJV)

My memory work in scripture has almost always been in the New King James Version of the Bible. It is quite poetic, and somehow easier for me to remember than some twentieth-century Bible translations.

Another passage of great importance to me is from the New Testament letter to the Ephesian Church.

He gave some, apostles; and some, prophets; and some, evangelists; and some, pastors and teachers; For the perfecting of the saints, for the work of the ministry, for the edifying of the body of Christ: Till we all come in the unity of the faith, and of the knowledge of the Son of God, unto a perfect man, unto the measure of the stature of the fullness of Christ. (Ephesians 4:11–13 NKJV)

God supplied all kinds of jobs for us—assigned us all a place of ministry—and in that work we find fullness of life. We find explanation of all that we cannot explain or understand in this life. It is in this mental state that we deal best with life's stresses and reduce the physiologic effects of out-of-control stress hormones.

The third scriptural passage of great value to me is from the first short letter of the Apostle Peter to the early church.

May the God of all grace, who called us to His eternal glory by Christ Jesus, after you have suffered a while, perfect, establish, strengthen, and settle you. To Him be the glory and the dominion forever and ever. Amen (1 Peter 5:10–11 NKJV)

Part of the equation of life for all God's children is suffering. It may be physical, sociologic, psychologic, financial, or otherwise, but it is all part of the perfecting process that matures human beings and gives meaning to our existence, which is often associated with struggles and life stresses.

This next scripture I share is a little like the others in that it also deals with that interesting work of perfecting. In New Testament Greek, the word *katartizo* is "to make perfect." This word is used often in the New Testament and is for me, in the Christian sense, what I am doing during my time here. It is a process—often associated with struggle, stress, and suffering—that ultimately produces a spiritually completed human being. This passage is from my favorite New Testament Scripture—the letter to the Hebrews—in the last few verses of that marvelous work.

Now may the God of Peace who brought up our Lord Jesus from the dead, that great Shepherd of the sheep, through the blood of the everlasting covenant, make you complete in every good work to do His will, working in you what is well pleasing in His sight, through Jesus Christ, to whom be glory forever and ever. Amen. (Hebrews 13:20–21 NKJV)

This verse taught me the ultimate way to deal with stress-related hormones. My commission was to pray and trust that He would dwell in me, abide in me, and take control of most of what I do. I began to pray for fewer choices in important things—less of me and more of Him, to allow God to move through my thoughts and actions. Trust is the substance of Christian faith and likely what pushed me to write this book.

I would be remiss, however, in not referencing one scripture that trumps all of the others in giving us a chance at good physical and spiritual health. The thirteenth chapter of the first letter to the Corinthian Church in the Christian New Testament basically says that even if I do everything I should do physically, mentally, and spiritually—if I do it all well but have no love—I am nothing. Selfless love trumps everything else. If we don't have it, we become as sounding brass and clanging cymbals, and our lives—though they may be rich and famous—are worthless in eternity.

If I speak in the tongue of men or of angels, but do not have love, I am only a resounding gong or a clanging cymbal. If I have the gift

of prophecy and can fathom all mysteries and all knowledge, and if
I have a faith that can move mountains, but do not have love, I am
nothing. If I give all I possess to the poor and give over my body to
hardship that I may boast, but do not have love, I gain nothing. (1
Corinthians 13:1–3 NKJV)

I trust that those who take the time to read this work will
reassess at this moment their own place in eternity and embrace
the love that comes only from God and intimacy with the Savior.
The end of the third chapter of the letter to the Ephesians and
the end of the eighth chapter of the letter to the Romans in the
New Testament say it best.

For this reason I bow my knees to the Father of our Lord Jesus
Christ, from whom the whole family in heaven and earth is named,
that He would grant you, according to the riches of His glory, to be
strengthened with might by His Spirit in the inner man, that Christ
may dwell in your hearts through faith; that you, being rooted and
grounded in love, may be able to comprehend with all the saints what
is the width and length and depth and height—to know the love of
Christ which passes all knowledge; that you may be filled with all
the fullness of God. (Ephesians 3:14–19 NKJV)

I am persuaded that neither death nor life, nor angels nor principal-
ities nor powers, nor things present nor things to come, nor height
nor depth, nor any other created thing shall be able to separate us
from the love of God which is in Christ Jesus our Lord. (Romans
8:38–39 NKJV)

Obviously, many reading this book are not particularly reli-
gious or perhaps have no belief in God or any deity. The basic
principles of spiritual health, however, cross all human bound-

aries. We all need to have a reason to exist—and simple ways to have a peaceful spirit and not be anxious, angry, fearful, or stressed. Reading great books, listening to lovely music, and enjoying beautiful sculptures and other art are all ways to have better spiritual health.

I am trusting and hopeful in Judeo-Christian ideas. Regardless of belief systems, I encourage all to spend time in activities that quiet your spirit and give you peace in your days—and in your nights.

PART FOUR

CHAPTER SIXTEEN

OPTIMAL HEALTH MAINTENANCE

WHAT CAN WE DO?

So, if we have perfect composition, perfect fitness, perfect nutrition, perfect spiritual health (a very challenging but rewarding prospect), perfect avoidance of toxins, perfect sleep, and wonderful health screening, what could possibly go wrong? In this chapter, I discuss—to the best of my ability— what goes wrong at a root level to lead to death.

Much of what I write will likely be proven to be in error. Some might lead to righteous criticism of an ancient physician for putting his late-in-life thoughts on paper. For my wrong presumptions, I apologize in advance. For ideas that stimulate new thoughts and lead to initiation of new practice patterns for physicians, I am preemptively grateful and this work will have been worth the effort. If you have read this far, you should have a pretty good idea of what I think goes wrong to lead to problems. This chapter ties it all together and offers a smooth transition for how we might change the course of healthcare. I hope you enjoy the ride.

THE AGING PROCESS

First, we need to acknowledge that most diseases that cause death in human beings do not begin in youth. The three main causes of death for the human community are accidents, vascular (cardiac) disease, and malignancies. All other diseases line up under these in terms of frequency. Young people have far fewer deaths than old people for all three main causes of death. The obvious conclusion is that aging must have something to do with death. If young people typically don't get a particular disease and old people do, it must be caused in some way by the aging process—or its consequence.

But what is it about aging that makes elderly people more likely to develop vascular disease or grow malignant tissue? We physicians try to understand associations for disease processes. For example, if we breathe smoke, we are more likely to develop lung cancer. The real question is why so many old people who smoke develop lung cancer, while most young people who smoke do not. If smoking also aggravates the atherosclerotic process in the arteries, why does smoking not do so in young people but does in those who are older? The same story goes for almost every chronic disease that causes death.

One might argue that these diseases are related to the duration of exposure. So, if I smoke for ten years, I probably won't get sick from it, but if I smoke for thirty years, I am more likely to get sick. This is likely true to some extent, but if a forty-year-old and sixty-year-old have both smoked for twenty years, the sixty-year-old has a much greater chance of dying of lung cancer than does the forty-year-old who has smoked the same number of cigarettes.

Something about the aging process enhances the likelihood of a bad outcome more so than in a younger person. What is it about aging that does this? What part of the aging process allows bad things to happen? I have wondered about this for years, but little is written specifically about this topic. Aging is said to cause a lot of negative health issues, and many ultimately result in disease and death.

Perhaps a better way to get to where I am going with this discussion is to ask my readers to pick which of the following organs or organ systems has the greatest likelihood—by itself—of causing aging and disease in other systems of the body? See what you come up with. Choose which of the following organ systems you believe is most likely to cause disease of itself or other organ systems as it gets older:

- Cardiovascular system
- Kidneys and urology system
- Lungs and pulmonary tissue system
- Skin and nails
- Bones and cartilage
- Sinuses and digestive tissue
- Immune system (white blood cells and antibodies)
- Nervous system (brain and spinal cord)
- Bone marrow (red blood cells, white blood cells, platelets)
- Liver, pancreas, and blood sugar control system (insulin and glucagon)

Think carefully about each system, and consider what you know about how they influence one another. Does aging of the cardiovascular system result in disease of other systems—or vice versa? It causes strokes and heart attacks, and may compromise blood flow to many organs. No doubt disease of the cardiovascular system can cause failure of other organ systems, but is this the most important system that influences the others? Does aging of the kidneys and urologic system result in damage to other systems? Failed kidneys certainly cause other systems to work poorly. Does aging of the immune system result in damage to other organ systems? If the immune system fails, we die of cancer or severe infections.

All systems influence one another, and end-stage damage of any or all of them can cause death. If I have to pick one system, however, whose aging process negatively influences all of the others, I have to go with the digestive system and sinuses.

This may be surprising, because we have spent the first couple of hundred pages of this book exploring the immune system, all of its wondrous ways, and its pitfalls. If you have paid careful attention, however, you have learned that while the immune system does a lot of damage, most diseases of immunity occur because the immune system was damaged or became dysfunctional as a result of its interfaces with *microorganisms living in the sinuses and bowels*. I believe that the basic aging process occurs in the sinuses, and the small and large bowels, and negatively influences all other body systems.

How does this happen? The following discussion and drawings represent my take on what happens inside the body as someone ages. The processes are variable from person to person because of genetic differences, but the basic process that occurs in all of us at variable rates of speed is aging of the tube.

AGING OF THE TUBE

The tube extends from the sinuses in the skull to the anus, which is usually about thirty-five feet away. The tube has two basic functions. One is to absorb nutrients that are important to life. The other is to keep out everything that is not supposed to be absorbed into the body.

The tube is constructed in a most marvelous way so that these two processes occur with some degree of success from the time of one's birth until death, which is usually many years later. My hypothesis—and certainly not my own exclusively—is that aging of the tube ultimately negatively influences all other body systems (listed above) and ultimately causes diseases in most of them. These diseases—all of which began with aging of the tube—then cause human beings to die.

Malignancy of the urinary bladder did not really begin in the bladder. Atherosclerosis of the coronary arteries and carotid arteries did not really begin in the arteries. Diseases of skin, cartilage, bones, and other tissues did not begin in those organs. All, I believe, began in the aging process of the gut and sinuses.

If this is true, then the ultimate treatment of malignancies, vascular disease, and all diseases of unknown cause is reversal of the aging processes of the sinuses, and large and small intestines—or the manipulation of microorganisms that populate the bowels.

Currently, treatment of most diseases is done by specialists who take care of skin, nerves, bones, cartilages, hearts, lungs, kidneys, livers, and other organ systems. I spent the best years of my life taking care of end-stage kidney disease, knowing full well none of the diseases were caused by the kidneys. I knew intuitively that the processes damaging the kidneys always started somewhere else—not in the kidneys. I didn't know where the disease started—I just knew the kidneys were not responsible for the disease.

The end-stage diseases of all organs are treated as if they begin in the organ itself—as if, heart disease begins in the heart, skin diseases like psoriasis begin in the skin, and lung diseases begin in the lungs. The truth is that almost no diseases of unknown cause begin in the organ that is being damaged. My contention is that almost all diseases begin in the tube, and until we learn to manage health of the tube, all diseases of all organ systems will continue to be of unknown cause. It's no wonder that, in my fifty years as a physician, atherosclerosis, malignancies of all kinds, and a host of other diseases still have no known cause. We need to do better!

Figure 2 graphically explains how the process occurs. The process is much more complex than my drawing depicts, but you will hopefully get the idea.

TUBE MICROANATOMY

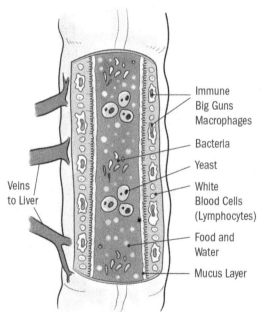

Figure 2.

As figure 2 depicts, the normal young tube is busy doing its jobs. It lets nutrients that are necessary for life get through the holes in the tube into tiny veins that drain from the bowel to the liver. The liver, which is a complex organ that performs more than three thousand known functions, takes the nutrients from the bowel and processes them into zillions of products that are necessary for life. Some of the blood goes on to endocrine organs that make hormones. Some goes to lymph tissue to make antibodies that enhance immunity, and so forth.

At the same time the tube is actively taking up nutrients through the holes in its lining, it is also in the process of keeping out things that are not intended to get into the blood vessels and go to the liver. This includes bacteria, fungi, protozoans, viruses, and other invaders, as well as chemicals made by the organisms. Millions of these little fellows grow luxuriantly in the tube. They make toxins and kill one another, and they eat the food we ingest and change it into various products through processes like fermentation. This is especially true of various carbohydrates we consume.

Amazingly, the holes in the tube—which allow good stuff to get in—are heavily guarded by elements of the immune system that do not allow bacteria, fungi, viruses, or protozoans to enter the tube lining. Even products these organisms make on a daily basis are mostly kept out of the bloodstream. The organisms do what they do every day inside the tube, but they do not enter the blood or mess with the body very much.

Once in a while, the tube becomes exposed to some new toxic germ. This includes all toxic bacteria that cause terrible diarrhea—cholera vibrio, salmonella, shigella, and various bad E. coli. These organisms are not part of the normal germs that live in the tube. They can cause invasion of the tube and terrible disease. In most cases of invasion by infectious organisms, strong antibiotics kill the invaders and allow normal life on the other side of the tube. Even in a person with a young tube, invasion by these kinds of organisms can be catastrophic. Thankfully, most are able to get well from such an invasion and return to a steady state in which the germs in the tube are back to normal activity and kept out of the depths of the tube's holes.

I believe life goes on pretty much normally for many years in our tubes. Nutrients come into the blood through the holes, and the immune system keeps bad stuff and any normal flora germs from getting very deep into the tube's holes. Humans live on the other side of the tube, pretty much ignoring what is going on in the tube. We eat food and sometimes pay a price for bad eating. We occasionally have allergies to various foods—when the immune system guarding the holes makes chemicals that go backward into our blood.

The soldiers of the immune system can make some pretty toxic substances themselves. They don't use their weapons often, but when they do, the immune system can make someone pretty sick pretty fast. In individuals who have allergies or sensitivities to foods, these immune activities are very bothersome. Such individuals have to be very careful of what they eat or their immune system will cause them to become very ill, and heroic medicines (adrenaline, cortisol, or others) may be required to save a life.

For the vast majority of individuals, however, there are no allergies or sensitivities, and daily life goes on normally. The germs live in the tube and do what they do. Healthy people live on the other side of the tube and do what they do. Everything is OK until a new process occurs in the tube. What is the process? Is it a malignancy or an infection? Is it an allergy to a particular food? Is it some hormone or nutrient deficiency? I don't believe so—at least not in most cases. What happens is—and there are no good tests to evaluate it—the tube gets older.

Yes, that's right. The tube gets older!

You might say, "That's the dumbest thing I have ever heard. Of course, the tube gets older. Everything gets older every day in every one of us. Who gives a dang if the tube gets older?"

The tube getting older is not quite the same as the arteries, kidneys, or gall bladder getting older. Most agree that aging skin doesn't look quite the same as it did in youth. Nothing about me is the same at age seventy-eight as it was when I was twenty. Everything is older. Oh, my skin still keeps out most of the invaders, but I've had recent skin cancers and keratoses I never had in the past. I still urinate, but my prostate gland and bladder don't do their jobs as well as they once did. My cartilages in my hands and feet never used to hurt, but they do now. I don't even smell or taste things as sharply as I used to.

None of this stuff is bad enough to keep me from getting out of bed, getting dressed, and going to work. All of it, however, is about getting older. Age-related dysfunction is common in many organ systems. But when the tube gets older, the prognosis is much more dire. Think about what the tube does. It lets good stuff in and keeps bad stuff out. It is the front door of the human body. It is well guarded, and it does its two jobs very well for a long time, assuming nutrition, fitness, sleep, and other functions are well managed. What do you think happens when the tube finally starts to fail?

Let's look at the tube in an older person and compare it with the tube of a young person. What is the obvious difference between the young tube and older tube? The old tube has bigger holes, and fewer immune system soldiers line the tubes. The big guns of the immune system still sit in readiness for invasion, but the tube as a whole does not look as formidable as it did when it was young. It looks more vulnerable, doesn't it?

YOUNG TUBE vs. OLD TUBE

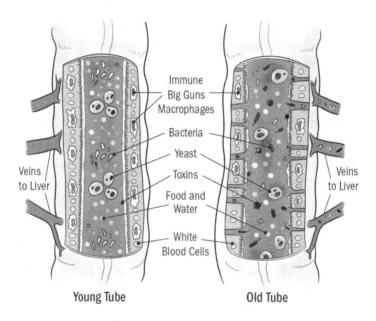

Young Tube

Old Tube

Immune Big Guns Macrophages

Bacteria

Yeast

Toxins

Food and Water

White Blood Cells

Veins to Liver

Veins to Liver

Figure 3.

In figure 4, notice the many microorganisms that live in the tube—around its holes, and in its hills and valleys. As you can see, there are even more per square inch of tube now than when the tube was young. Perhaps it's a population explosion— or maybe it's just that the immune soldiers have grown more comfortable with the germs and are putting up with more than was acceptable in the twenty-year-old tube.

OLD TUBE

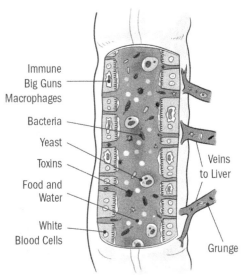

Immune
Big Guns
Macrophages

Bacteria

Yeast

Toxins

Food and
Water

White
Blood Cells

Veins
to Liver

Grunge

Figure 4.

Unfortunately, we cannot easily identify the subtle changes the aging process causes in the tube. If you look down the esophagus with an endoscope or look up into the colon with the longer colonoscope, the bowel lining looks much like it did when it was young. At a microscopic level, however, it is likely a much different story. The gaps between lining cells are enlarged. Often an increased layer of mucous is produced by white blood cells lining and coating the tube. The mucous blocks absorption of many key nutrients and also protects some microorganisms from digestive juices and acid that would ordinarily keep the growth of intestinal microorganisms at a low level. Because the holes get larger, the number of bacteria, yeast, viruses, and protozoans increases dramatically. It all looks the same as usual from a distant vantage point, but down in the trenches where the action is, a battle for life is taking place.

Remember that the organisms often make very toxic stuff that kills other organisms and would kill us if it were absorbed through the gut lining into the blood. Some of this toxin can now be measured in the blood. The commercially available lab test gauges levels of endotoxin or lipopolysaccharide (LPS).

As the aging process goes on and the war gets more heated, the holes continue to get larger and leak more toxins. This is the basis for leaky gut syndrome, shown in figure 5.

Fortunately, the highly trained immune system sits ready to suppress the age-induced invasion of yeast, bacteria, viruses, and toxins produced in the war against the human host. As this process gains momentum—either because of too many microorganisms per square inch or extra-large holes in the tube—the body calls on elements of the immune system that were previously not needed.

OLD TUBE BACTERIAL INVASION

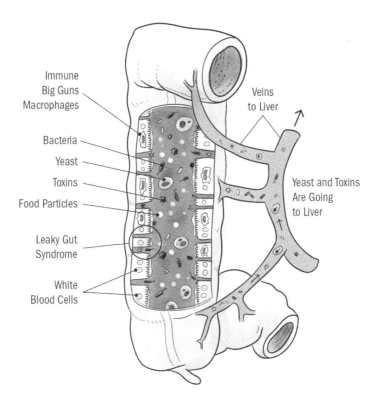

Figure 5.

The foot soldiers who stood at the front door of the holes in the tube for many years are now overwhelmed by the invaders. Toxins made by the microorganisms are getting deeper into the holes, and some of the toxins (LPS and organic acids) are getting into the blood—and will eventually show up in the urine. When this process occurs, a big-time response from the immune system is desperately needed.

Sitting at the back of the tube holes, as shown in figures 5 and 6, are the big guys of the immune system—the Sherman tanks and surface-to-air missiles, if you will—ready to save us from the invasion. These pieces of our immune system are wonderful in their capacity to kill germs and inactivate the toxins they make. The names of these tanks and missiles are numerous, including interleukin-6 interferon, tumor necrosis factor, and others—all stronger chemicals than the toxins made by the invaders.

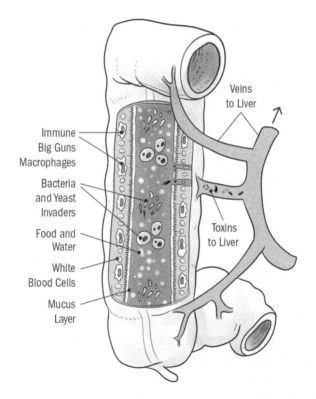

Figure 6.

As depicted in figure 6, during the early skirmishes of this battle, the microorganisms are easily kept at bay by these strong members of the immune system and by white blood cells and antibodies made in the tube's lymph system. We should indeed stand and cheer at the strength and depth of the immune system. It is a beautiful thing to behold. Although the aging process makes the holes bigger, and the mucous layer allows for the production of more invaders per square inch of tube, the fully alert immune system is more than ready to deal with the crisis. The invaders are driven back, and the toxins are destroyed. Who says aging is so bad anyway?

Not so fast! I should mention that activation of the so-called tanks and missiles at the back of the tube holes is not without a cost. As the missiles are fired and destroy the invaders, the missiles and tanks make combustion products. These products of war are released into the blood, which is on its way to the liver. As figure 6 shows, the LPS toxins from the germs in the tube get into the blood to some small extent, but there is even more of the discharge products from the tanks and missiles than there is toxin from the bacteria and yeast in the tube.

In layperson's language, the body is bombarded by products of the germs to some extent but by its own immune system products to an even larger extent. Figure 6 attempts to show this process. The liver is sitting uphill from these events, receiving blood from the bowel, and this complex organ in turn has to get ready for the onslaught of toxins. Lymph nodes along the way to the liver may filter some of the toxins, but finally the liver, which is like a huge lake full of veins, must go into action to keep the bad stuff from getting past it and into the blood that goes out to every part of the body. Thankfully, most people have good livers that can put up with a lot of poisoning and detoxify much of what comes from the gut.

Aging sets the stage, and the bacteria and yeast in the bowel take advantage of what aging does to the tube. The microorganisms make toxins that further poison the tube and get into the holes in the wall of the tube. The immune system goes to work to inactivate the organisms and detoxify the stuff made by the germs. We who own the tubes typically have no idea any of this is going on. We just look in the mirror and see our faces getting older, but we forget our tubes are getting older as well. It's one thing to have an old face—it's entirely another to have an old tube.

I hope you can see by now that the consequences of our having an old tube are significant. A dermatologist can cut the basal cell carcinoma from my cheek, but there is no "ologist" to repair the aging process in my tube. The tube just gets older, and depending upon my genetics, the war in my aging tube can cause a bevy of bad stuff to happen. Let's look at the next set of drawings to see what happens in several different individuals of varying genetic makeups when the battle is unfolding.

INFLUENCE OF GENETIC MAKEUP

As you can see in the next drawings, we have a husband and wife, Mary and Bill, who have been married for nearly forty years—eating the same stuff, going to the same movie theaters, and raising the same children. Both are sixty years old. Both have aging tubes, and both of them are totally unaware their tubes are getting older.

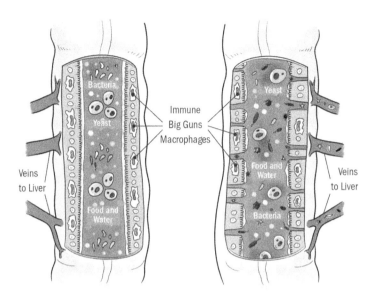

Figure 7.

Mary comes from a family whose members get atherosclerotic vascular disease as they mature. Bill's family members have died of mostly malignancies and autoimmune diseases in their older years. Mary's family has had some skin cancers but no internal malignancies. As shown in figure 7, both Mary and Bill have enlarged holes in their tubes, and they both face an onslaught of toxins made by their tube germs and some invasion of tube holes by microorganisms.

In this hypothetical model, let's say all of the organisms are bacteria and no fungi (candida) are in the tube. This is quite unlikely, since all of us have some fungus in our tubes. Bill and Mary have not taken many antibiotics during their lives, so they have mostly common bacteria like E. coli and Klebsiella growing in their tubes. As figure 8 shows, the microorganisms in the tube's holes are getting close enough to the tube blood going to the liver (portal vein blood) that they are causing the immune system's Sherman tanks and missiles to become activated.

BILL'S AGING TUBE

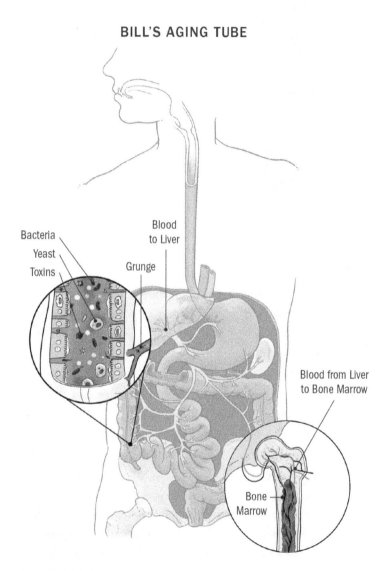

Figure 8.

These big guns are of various types and have a variety of names, as noted before. They do a good job of killing germs that are getting too close for comfort. Unfortunately, every time a surface-to-air missile is released at the back of the tube hole, the tank and missile launcher also release into the blood some products of immune system combustion, if you will—some pretty toxic stuff. These biochemical products—shown in figures 8 and 9, as black smoke clouds—are released into the blood going to the liver. This occurs hour after hour, as long as the invaders are entering the holes in the tube—that is, as long as the microorganisms are present.

As this occurs, all the toxic stuff released by activity of the immune system goes straight to the liver, where some of it is metabolized and converted to nontoxic products. Some of it, however, escapes unchanged from the liver and gets out into the blood. Such chemicals were never intended to get into people's blood. They are as foreign to Bill and Mary as some food they have never eaten. As is shown in figure 9, some of the chemicals released back into the gut from the surface-to-air missile launching pad are now going to unique places in the body.

Just for fun—and to help me make a point—let's name the chemicals "grunge." As you can see in figure 8, some grunge in Bill's blood is going to his immune-competent white blood cells in his bone marrow. As this grunge becomes attached to Bill's white cells (lymphocytes), some of these cells become damaged and lose their capacity to make important protective chemicals. One of the chemicals produced by lymphocytes is currently called tumor necrosis factor, which our lymphocytes produce all of the time during health. As long as Bill's white blood cells are capable of making this chemical, he is protected against growing malignant tumor cells.

When grunge from the gut is present, however, Bill's white blood cells can't make much of the tumor necrosis factor. This in turn allows cancer cells to form in Bill's pancreas, prostate gland, or another organ. Sadly, toxins coming from the microorganisms in the tube. or the products made by the tanks and surface-to-air missiles, are sufficient to damage the white blood cells (lymphocytes) that make the tumor necrosis factor. The result is that Bill begins to develop a tumor in one or more of his important organs. Bill's aging gut has set in motion processes that might lead to his developing a malignant tumor at some location in his body.

If this happens, he will likely see a gastroenterologist, urologist, or other specialist who takes care of tumors of the pancreas, prostate gland, or other internal organs. These doctors will give Bill some chemotherapy to kill his tumors—and they will hopefully be successful for a time—but ultimately the toxins coming from the organisms in the gut or the chemicals made by the big guns of the immune system in the tube will ultimately lead to Bill's death from cancer.

Physicians who take care of Bill's cancer have no idea why the tumor developed in his pancreas, prostate gland, or other organ. They treat the end organ that is diseased and the complications of the disease, paying no attention to what really caused the problems—which are, of course, in progress in the aging tube. A number of medicines advertised on television are anti-tumor-necrosis medicines—they inactivate this important chemical—and we get to hear the forty-five-second disclaimer about the risk of cancer if you take this medicine to treat your psoriasis, Crohn's, or whatever.

Mary has an entirely different genetic family background than her husband's, but has generally the same germs growing in her tube as her husband does. Her tube is aging in the same way as Bill's. Her holes are getting larger. She has more organisms per square inch than she had when she was young. She is, therefore, developing leaky gut syndrome, as more toxic products get absorbed into her tube blood on its way to her liver. Mary's big guns are being activated, and grunge is being produced by Mary's Sherman tanks and surface-to-air missiles. The grunge gets into her blood and goes to her liver, where much of it is metabolized and inactivated. Some of it, however, gets into her blood as it flows through the liver and out to the rest of her body. As with her husband, some of Mary's grunge gets attached to her white blood cells that make the tumor necrosis factor.

Mary, however, has good genetic resistance to this type of damage. She, therefore, does not suffer any deficiency of her tumor necrosis factor. As depicted in figure 9, she does not develop tumors in her pancreas, liver, or other organs. Mary's excess grunge, however, goes to some other places that are important to her future health. As figure 9 shows, her grunge goes to the intimal linings of her carotid, coronary, and other arteries all over her body. In these locations, grunge from the gut causes local irritation and inflammation, which create the beginning of what may become atherosclerotic plaquing of her arteries in these and other locations. This process goes on for quite a while before the atherosclerotic plaques are sufficiently large to result in poor blood supply to her heart, brain, and other organs.

Both Bill and Mary, in these simple examples, are exposed to the same grunge coming from the discharge of the surface-to-air missile launcher in the immune system of the gut. The potential outcomes for each of them are very different, however. The greater the invasion of the holes in the gut lining, the greater likelihood that the big guns of the immune system will be activated and make grunge that gets into the blood—for both Bill and Mary.

MARY'S AGING TUBE

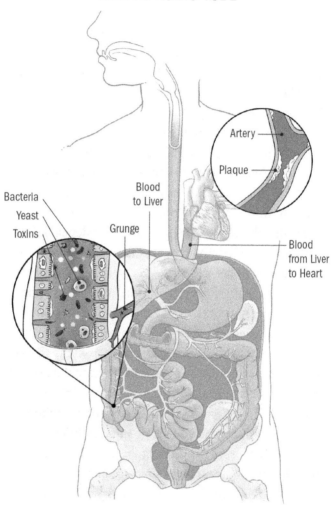

Figure 9.

The cause of the entire problem for each of them is aging of the tube, whose aging immune system can no longer control the advancing invasion of normal microorganisms of the gut. Bill and Mary each experience a unique response to the increased production of grunge in the gut, very much related to genetic handling of the poison. Mary's grunge results in her risk of developing vascular disease in the intimal linings of her arteries. Bill's grunge messes up his immune surveillance system for cancer prevention. His grunge does nothing to the linings of his arteries, but causes him to be at risk of developing a malignancy. Mary's grunge poisons the linings of her arteries and can result in plaque disease. It's a demonstration of one common starting point with two very different prospective endings.

Who will Mary and Bill see in the healthcare system for treatment of their illnesses? Mary will see a cardiologist or vascular surgeon. Bill will see a gastroenterologist, urologist, or oncologist. None will correctly diagnose the real cause of the problem.

REVIEWING THE POSSIBILITIES

I hope my readers see the potential for truth in my hypothetical scenarios. In neither case was there an infection, but the entire process was nevertheless caused by germs as they complicated the aging process of the tube. This is not a disease of the tube, like Crohn's disease or ulcerative colitis. It is simply the normal aging process—with the possible end result being vascular disease in one person and cancer in the other.

Knowing the processes are in progress and with a good test for tube function, what should be the approach to treat the patient? Only two basic choices come to the rational mind:

1. Kill some of the microorganisms so there are not so many invading the holes in the tube.
2. Change the holes in the tube, or make them smaller and less vulnerable to bacteria and yeast invasion.

Either of these should reverse the process and prevent Bill and Mary from developing malignancy and vascular diseases. Unfortunately, neither Bill nor Mary knew early in the process that anything at all was wrong with them. As far as each could tell, their tube was working perfectly. Aging was doing a number on both of them, and they would both potentially end up with diseases that annually kill millions of people worldwide.

Of course, many variables could change the abovementioned processes and outcomes. Increased production of mucous in the aging bowel may increase the number of organisms present per square inch in the tube of either Bill or Mary. This by itself, even without much aging, could lead to increased invasion of the tube holes and ultimately the production of grunge. Bill and Mary's doctors could try to measure grunge levels, but such measurements are not routinely done in current medical communities. We can now measure blood LPS levels or urinary organic acids, but for the most part, physicians do not yet measure these toxic bacterial products.

This story could also be written around different environmental variables for both characters. A change in diet for Bill or Mary could lead to new patterns of microorganisms in the bowels and change what was going on in the immune systems of their tubes. Either or both of them could take a course of antibiotics for treatment of a sinus or urinary infection that would cause production of increased amounts of candida or other yeasts in their tubes. In general, I favor not having much yeast in my bowel and hoping for colonization with mainly good bacteria.

For now, we simply need to acknowledge that aging causes all tissues to change. As I look down at my seventy-eight-year-old skin, I see a very different look than I saw when I was twenty-seven years old. While my skin does not have any named diseases at this moment, it appears to be very scarred, bruised, thin, and vulnerable. I'm sure every organ in my body has some changes. Fortunately, all my organs seem to still work pretty well, but they are all vulnerable to damaging influences that come from other locations—like the tube.

It is my contention that aging of the gut trumps all other aging processes, because the war for our lives takes place in the lining of the tube. We die of heart disease, malignancies of various organs, strokes, immunologic diseases, and diseases of unknown cause. None of these processes, however, kills on the day it begins to happen. The process that causes a stroke, heart attack, or malignancy has likely been operative for many months or years before a major clinical event occurs. The processes are relentless, however, because the war in the tube is relentless.

I could share countless stories of folks like Bill and Mary who offer variations of the same story. Depending on genetics, organs damaged by tube disease can be quite diverse. The genetics of the immune system lining the tube, and the immune system that protects from malignant disease, is likely quite diverse from person to person. In my kidney and heart transplant experiences with HLA typing (forty different A and B tissue types), I've seen immeasurable amounts of variables in immune appearances of different individuals. Different genetics lead to different outcomes from a single process in the aging tube.

The same process going on in the gut can result in psoriasis and psoriatic arthritis in one person and rheumatoid arthritis in another. One person with a different HLA type could suffer the same insult and end up with vasculitis or some other terrible disease of unknown cause. The possibilities of different end-organ diseases related to these processes are nearly endless.

This is why pathology textbooks are so thick and heavy, and why so many medical and surgical subspecialists are taking care of all our diseases. It is why we spend countless dollars on cardiac research and cancer research, and still have astronomical death rates from malignancies and vascular disease. We will never run out of genetic variations on this theme. Family disease will segregate along genetic lines, and family history can loosely predict what might cause someone to die.

Nevertheless, if we go back to the true cause of all these diseases, health management becomes much clearer. To win the game, we must learn to manipulate what goes on in the tube. In the few remaining pages of this writing, I formulate some ideas regarding tube management. It seems to be the only hope in reducing the complexity of medicine and the exorbitant costs of healthcare.

CHAPTER SEVENTEEN

MANAGING THE TUBE

Tube management is essentially about recognition that the mucosal surface of the mouth, sinuses, and bowels is an ever-changing environment. Microorganisms that live on the surface influence the health of those of us who live on the other side of the tube. Even if we practice perfect health, the natural aging of the tube can create all sorts of medical problems. This ties into the two premises stated at the beginning of the book, summarized here:

Toxins made by the organisms can enter the gut blood and cause disease. Other chemicals (grunge) made by the immune system in response to the organisms, can also enter gut blood and cause disease.

I suspect that most chronic human disease is caused by these two processes. If we wish to stay as healthy as possible or recover well from illnesses, a great part of good, overall health is learning how to manage the tube. Of course, this is not necessarily as simple as it sounds.

I would be lying if I were to tell you I am an expert in tube management. If you were to ask me to send you to see a good tube manager, I would likely draw a blank and tell you I don't know of anyone nearby. Healthcare directories do not have sections that point to good tube managers. Index entries under "physicians and surgeons" in computer databases do not detail any tube managers. The reason for this is there are no official tube managers.

My gastroenterology friends are experts in diagnosis and treatment of gastrointestinal diseases like Crohn's disease, ulcerative colitis, and irritable bowel syndrome, and patients are very grateful for what they do. Nevertheless, even they do not go into great depth looking into the aging processes in the bowel. Currently, there are no tests to tell whether bowel function is old, young, or middle aged.

Tube management must reside, in the years ahead, with those who believe my theory and then apply various management tools to deal with the aging process in the bowel. This will require creativity and courage, since it will likely be some time before the medical world recognizes the nature of the problem.

I suspect this area of medicine will be recognized first in the offices of primary care physicians who are willing to step out on a limb and try new therapies designed to reverse some pathologic issues. I have my own ideas of what can be done to cope with the aging process in the bowel, and I address those in this chapter. I hope my ideas will be valuable to some and will improve the quality of life for many who read this volume.

If the fundamental problem with an aging bowel is some combination of bacterial and yeast overgrowth, and a tube that has larger than normal holes for absorption of bowel contents, then management of the problem is either to heal the tube, reduce the size of the holes, or reduce the number of invading bacteria or yeast. But how can we heal the tube when we don't even know for sure the tube needs to be healed?

This is a very difficult question with several possible answers.

THE DEVELOPMENT OF URINE TESTING
FOR GUT MICROFLORA

Sometime in the late 1980s, when I was still practicing nephrology but also beginning to develop an executive examination program as well as a nutrition and obesity management enterprise, my eyes came upon an ad from a laboratory in Atlanta, Georgia. The lab had a urine test that reportedly analyzed amounts of various organic acids in the urine of patients with various diseases and correlated the urinary levels of these chemicals with disease symptoms.

What caught my eye was the notation that none of these organic acids in the urine was human organic acid. They were all organic acids produced in the gut by bacteria and yeast. The physicians managing the lab suggested the amounts of these organic acids had strong correlations with the presence of immune diseases in the patients who had produced the urine. In those early urine specimens, the physicians found organic acids from aerobic bacteria, anaerobic bacteria, and yeast, and determined normal ranges for each of the organic acids. The test could only tell the amounts of organic acids per unit volume of urine. All the test told for sure was that there was stuff in the urine that had no business being in the urine of a healthy adult. The only location where such acids could be made in volume was in the gut, by the microorganisms that live there.

I ordered a number of those urine studies back in the 1980s and 1990s. It was amazing how many patients with elevated levels of the organic acids were sick with headaches, coughs, irritable bowel syndrome, eczema, psoriasis, and arthritis. Sometimes the organic acid elevations came from bacteria and others were made by yeast. All the organic acids were made in the gut, absorbed into the blood, and filtered into the urine by the kidneys.

The question the lab physicians could not answer was whether or not the presence of elevated levels of these organic acids was caused by too many organisms per square inch of bowel or some disease of the bowel. The latter came to be known as leaky gut syndrome.

TUBE TESTING

The simplest answer to gauging tube function would be to measure something in the blood or urine that suggests whether or not the tube is leaking. Good testing tells us if something is wrong—for example, if a patient is likely being poisoned from the tube—and that balance in the tube needs to be restored, perhaps it's with treatment such as Pepto Bismol, antibiotics, probiotics, nutrients, aloe vera, or other medicines that become available for changing bowel flora and preventing poisons. Clinical measurements lead to better therapy. Right now, we don't even know when poisoning is happening, and it likely goes on for a long time before we know we have been poisoned.

Simple tests to poisoning by gut microflora *are* available, such as the measurement of blood lipopolysaccharide levels (LPS)—which is a commercially available test at this time—or organic acids made by bacteria or yeast that are present in the urine—also a test that is commercially available in several laboratories.

The urine test for gut microflora has been available for two decades, but most physicians have never heard of it and therefore have not requested it for their patients. If I as a physician knew my patient had elevated urinary levels of these organic acids or elevated blood levels of LPS, I would be much more likely to initiate therapy designed to change the tube or manipulate the microorganisms at the root of the problem.

The problem with this type of testing is that not many doctors are doing it, so the normal range for measurements can be difficult to determine. As an experienced physician, I hate to initiate new kinds of testing or treatment on people who are seeing other physicians. We physicians are essentially members of a club that has high standards and expects all club members to play by the rules. Using new types of testing or therapies is somewhat of a risk for those who want continued membership in the club.

That being said, the desire to have well patients sometimes demands that we enter into informal clinical trials of diagnostic tests and therapies that are a little out of the mainstream. Drawing a blood test for LPS is not harmful to patients—nor is collecting a urine specimen to check for bacterial or fungal organic acids. It isn't harmful, but it is not commonly done. I suspect that twenty years from now, all physicians will routinely obtain this kind of testing on patients.

THE SHOTGUN APPROACH

The other approach to the aging gut as a source of pathology takes more faith and less science, but it can yield remarkable results from time to time. The thinking in this case goes something like this: A patient comes to the doctor's office with a new complaint. The complaint has no obvious cause, and the doctor has to surmise what might be causing the problem. The doctor asks a few questions and perhaps does a brief physical examination pertinent to the patient's symptoms. At the end of this encounter, the physician has to make an educated guess as to what is most likely causing the patient's symptoms and what might be done to make things better.

If the illness remains a mystery, the physician might punt and tell the patient it must be some kind of virus, or that the patient may have a stress-related syndrome. We can chuckle at such thinking, but this is sometimes what goes on when physicians are confronted with unusual symptoms.

In such a situation, what would you think if the physician were to say the following to you? "Mrs. Smith, I suspect your immune system is causing your symptoms. You have a variant of an allergic reaction. I'm not sure what is causing the allergic reaction, and we may not be able to find out right away. We may have to make an educated guess. If the allergic reaction is caused by some chemical in your environment—like soap, perfume, or household cleaner—we of course want you to stop that exposure.

"If, however, the allergic reaction is caused by an immune response to bacteria or yeast in your bowel or sinuses, we have no way of knowing if a problem of this type exists. If we knew you were having an allergic reaction to bacteria or yeast, we would of course want to kill the bacteria or yeast. We have good medicines that do this. We also have a few good medicines that can safely shut down your immune system for a few days—so we can see whether your immune system is indeed responsible for your symptoms. We could give you medicine to shut off the allergy, but if the allergy is in response to a microorganism like a yeast or bacterium, we would want to kill this germ while suppressing the allergy."

This would depend, of course, on the degree of discomfort induced by the allergy in a given patient and other unique circumstances. Many patients may be willing to try a shotgun approach to their disease to suppress immunity with steroids and kill unknown germs with antibiotics and nystatin or another antifungal agent.

In my experience as a physician who has taken care of dreadfully ill patients, most people are willing to try new therapies if the simple things they have already tried are not working—and, of course, if the risks of taking corticosteroids and antibiotics do not seem too great. The amazing thing to me is that so very many patients have a positive response to this approach. It is certainly outside the mainstream of medicine—and there are some small risks. In my opinion, however, the potential benefits far outweigh the risks in most cases. If there is a possibility that germs are causing the disease through interaction with the immune system, I believe the treatment of choice should be to kill the germs.

MAKING THE TUBE YOUNG AGAIN

Tools for making old tubes young again are somewhat limited. Dietary fiber, probiotics, prebiotics, Pepto Bismol, aloe vera, garlic extract, corticosteroids, and a host of micronutrients all have a place in tube management. The mainstay of therapy, however, at the present time is management of the microorganisms that grow in the tube.

Good therapy of difficult health problems may involve reducing the total number of organisms per square inch of bowel surface or changing the entire nature of what is growing in the tube at the time. Clearly, yeast organisms grow better when we kill certain bacteria, and many bacteria grow better when we kill yeast.

But as I have said often, it is difficult to change the total nature of what is growing in the tube. It's like throwing mud balls at a wallpapered wall. It takes a lot of mud to hide the wallpaper. In the same way, it may take months of antibiotic suppression to make a significant change in microflora. The story of my patient with rheumatoid arthritis early in this writing attests to the occasional need for long-term use of antibiotics to change the organisms that cause chronic cartilage pain and swelling.

CONCLUSION

I t has taken me seventeen chapters to say what I feel needed to be said about the causes of disease. I have been privileged to care for some of the sickest people in the world and have been blessed to learn from them. My proposed approach to disease may not work for you or me with our infirmities, but my experiences with hundreds of patients tell me the benefits of such an approach far outweigh the risks in most cases.

The big question is whether or not we physicians have the courage to be creative in our thinking and try new ideas in the management of old problems. All forces of academia, the pharmaceutical industry, the insurance industry, and the legal profession are aligned against such thinking. Unfortunately, healthcare is at the present time much like everything else in society. If you want to know where it's going, just follow the money.

Treatment of vascular disease with ten dollars a month for antibiotics, antifungal agents, and nutrients sounds like an unlikely therapeutic possibility when the standard of care at the present time includes coronary artery bypass, angioplasty, statin medicines, immunosuppressive drugs, and a host of new chemicals that decrease blood cholesterol levels. It's no wonder I am finishing fifty years of medicine, and the same diseases that caused death and destruction when I entered the field are still of unknown cause—and still causing death and destruction. It is indeed a tragedy.

I firmly believe it's time to change that. So where do we go from here? Keep reading to learn what I feel is the best shot at family physicians and other creative clinicians moving toward functional medicine.

TREAT THE UNDERLYING CAUSE

If many of the diseases that cause human beings to get sick and die are strongly related to gut bacteria and yeast, or the immunologic response to bacteria or yeast in an aging bowel, we ought to expect our physicians to choose therapies that are the least expensive and least toxic. If many chronic illnesses emanate from the biome of the gut and the immune response to the biome, other diseases likely have the same cause.

But how do we know if the problem is caused by yeast or bacteria—or both—in any given clinical situation? My experiences over the years give me a rough idea of which organisms might cause which kinds of diseases, but I admit I often don't know the answer to the question and simply have to proceed with a shotgun approach to therapy.

Sadly, until we routinely make use of urine studies of bacterial or fungal organic acids, we may not have a very good idea which type of organism is at the root of the problem. If there is no clear-cut known relationship between the disease and which germs may be causing it, killing both bacteria and yeast may be necessary as a trial. Thankfully, we have safe antibiotics and antifungal drugs that have few side effects, to use in a shotgun approach.

That being said, my experiences tell me certain disease conditions seem to be more likely related to allergic reactions to yeast than to bacteria. I believe most asthma is likely related to yeast growth in the bowel. Some cases, like those of my dialysis clinic patients who got better with nystatin, apparently had yeast as the cause of chronic cough. Clearly, one patient who had asthma got a lot better when I gave her a medicine that killed yeast in the bowel. Apparently either yeast in the bowel—or bacteria in the bowel or airway, as per Dr. Hahn's excellent work—in selected individuals may result in the clinical picture of asthma.

However, based on data referenced previously, if microorganisms are indeed the instigators of coronary and other vascular disease, then the likely culprits are bacterial and not fungal. Psoriasis, rheumatoid arthritis, and other types of cartilage disease are likely related to immunologic reactions to gut bacteria. Joint pain and eye diseases (iritis and scleritis) associated with ulcerative colitis and inflammatory bowel disease are likely bacterial in genesis.

With nearly one thousand different species of bacteria growing in the bowel, the numbers of unique disease presentations could be very vast. I suspect many more diseases said to be autoimmune begin in the bowel as the immune system deals with what is going on in the tube. Systemic lupus, based on my experiences, could well be related to an immunologic reaction to yeast in the bowel. My experiences tell me fungi like candida are likely at the root of fibromyalgia and chronic fatigue—terribly debilitating muscle weakness syndromes that have decreased the quality of many lives.

Yeast is likely the culprit in various types of eczema involving skin in various parts of the body. Chronic middle ear symptoms with fluid behind the tympanic membrane can sometimes be treated by killing yeast in the bowel. Some types of chronic pain seem to be aggravated in some way by immunologic reactions to yeast. If we don't eliminate the yeast, we don't get to find out whether or not there is improvement in pain had we killed some yeast—in the tube or elsewhere.

My experience with recurrent cedar pollen allergies suggests that killing or suppressing bowel yeast can lead to an enormous improvement in allergy symptoms in some people. Killing yeast isn't high on the to-do list for allergists, but I suspect it should be. The list of diseases related to microorganisms could go on and on. The important mental process for a physician is, "Could this condition be caused by or aggravated by the presence of a certain group of bacteria or yeast?"

Often the answer would be, "I don't know." If the answer is "possibly," then a trial of antibacterial or antifungal therapy might be in order.

RECIPE FOR FUNCTIONAL TREATMENT

If I were to write a recipe that best describes my recommendation for taking care of illness, based upon the data detailed in this book, it would go something like this:

1. Let's say you develop a new bothersome symptom that suggests something is out of balance in your body. Obviously, if you were involved in some trauma, you would likely blame the trauma for the symptom. If no cause, however, is obvious, ask this: "Might germs have anything to do with my symptom or set of symptoms?"
2. The next question would be, "Am I missing something from

my environment or diet that is causing this symptom or set of symptoms?"

3. Next, ask yourself, "Is there anything I am doing or eating that could be causing this symptom or set of symptoms?"

4. Depending upon the acuteness and severity of your symptoms, you might at this time consider trying some over-the-counter remedy to treat symptoms: aspirin, ibuprofen, Pepto Bismol, Imodium, decongestants, acetaminophen, diphenhydramine, or any of dozens of different creams or lotions.

5. If your symptoms continue, worsen, or expand in number, entertain the possibility that all your symptoms are related to some underlying process, and that germs and the immune system's response to germs may be operative.

6. The next question would logically be, "Which germs might be causing the problem that is resulting in my symptoms?" Could it be fungi, bacteria, virus, protozoan organisms interfacing with the immune system in the sinuses, mouth, bowel, vaginal wall, or skin?

7. This is where I suggest that you might seek a creative and courageous physician who would consider recommending a course of trial therapy to include antibiotics, antifungal agents, antiviral agents, and possibly a Medrol Dosepak or two to shut off the distorted immunity. If the steroids cause a reduction in your symptoms over the first few days of medication, the antibiotics chosen should be continued for days to weeks to see if improvement in your symptoms is sustained. If symptom improvement is sustained, the only question left is, "How long should my physician continue prescribing the antibiotics?"

8. As noted, nystatin—because it is not absorbable—can be continued for months to years without any negative side

effects. Antibiotics, which are absorbed into your blood, can often be taken for long periods of time—but with humble caution. Nevertheless, the long-term goal for this kind of therapy should be elimination of all prescription drugs when your clinical problem has resolved—or when you and your physician know for sure that the trial of medications was not effective and that another approach is warranted.

9. You might try the regimen, under your doctor's supervision, with several different antibiotics until it is determined your disease or condition is unresponsive to therapy, and that some unexplained and still unknown process is operative.

10. Along the way, you might try some dietary changes—like those discussed in the books *The Yeast Connection* or *Eat Right 4 Your Type*. Remember that simple maneuvers like change in dietary components can often cause profound changes in the types of bacteria or yeast growing in your bowels, sinuses, and other mucous membranes.

11. A more sophisticated approach might include measurement of IgG antibodies to foods—available from some national laboratories at a cost of several hundred dollars. For some patients, this may be a minimal cost for a large gain in clinical information—and sometimes resolution of complex symptoms.

The above recommendations represent a new way of thinking about clinical problems for patients and their primary care physicians—and for many specialty physicians as well.

As I review the medical literature, I clearly see that each decade brings a host of newly named diseases, which are identified by more and more sophisticated technology. This results in new disease specialties with new tests and new costs, ultimately leading to patients going to various different physicians for care. This has to stop somewhere, especially when it becomes apparent that almost all the pathology begins with very simple processes that might be aborted with simple changes in diet, simple antibiotic regimens, and simple anti-inflammatory medicines.

If I were to start over and become a family physician committed to the total care of people, I would want just a very few medicines in my black bag. I would want a couple of blood pressure medicines to deal with elevated pressures that are refractory to changes in patient behavior. I would want three or four different antibiotics that could kill a variety of different kinds of bacteria in the sinuses, ears, skin, and bowels. I would want some nystatin and fluconazole to treat fungi growing in the sinuses and bowel. Finally, I would want a few bottles of Medrol or prednisone to help patients with suppression of inflammatory activity. My bet is that with this small black bag of simple and inexpensive medicines, I could make a lot of people get a lot better much of the time. Oh yes—I would also want to throw in a few bottles of aspirin and some Pepto Bismol for tube management and suppression of inflammation.

I'm only sorry I was not taught these principles in medical school or during my residency and fellowship training. They would have made me a better physician and likely would have saved a number of lives—and a great deal of money and inconvenience engendered by an out-of-control healthcare system.

MEDICINE OF THE FUTURE

No doubt health begins, first and foremost, with us. We must all work to maintain good body composition. We all need good muscles and bones, and not excessive amounts of stored fat. Remember also that, to a good extent, we are what we eat and therefore must be more expert at choosing foods that help us and don't hurt us or cause us to die early. Physical fitness is also vital, and we should embrace the benefits of activity in general.

A lot of print space in this book points to the problem of poisoning, which in essence is what we are trying to avoid by managing the tube. Remember that the world is full of other poisons—combustion products, ethyl alcohol, and prescription drugs of various kinds lead the way. Staying away from such poisons promotes sustained health, as does moderating stress through good sleep and exposure to spiritual health disciplines that allow joy, peace, patience, kindness, goodness, gentleness, and other qualities associated with longevity. All these are important if we hope to live long, healthy, productive lives.

But once the aging process takes over, some changes in the body that lead to ill health might be unpreventable. Knowing the importance of the tube and managing it to the best of your ability can help you be stronger and more vital for longer. I hope the information in this book empowers you to better understand your body and take a measure of control over your health. Consider talking to your doctors about it, like the patient who spoke with me about Dr. Crook's *The Yeast Connection*.

I extend God's richest blessings to all who took the time to read this book. I pray my writing will help many get well from difficult illnesses of unknown cause and will inspire courage in some of my primary care colleagues who are tired of sending patients down the road to a myriad of specialists. Medicine of the future must be far less expensive and less toxic than it is currently. We can do better!

When I began this writing, I was bemoaning the clutter of my television screen with new drug commercials. Sadly, these continue to increase in numbers with little evidence that they are going away anytime soon. Some of these drugs are likely a blessing to many, but they are expensive and often toxic—and they typically treat symptoms without solving what causes most diseases. My best hope is that tube care becomes a major part of health and wellness programs of the next generation. In a nation being torn apart by the cost of and provision of good healthcare, tube care could make a huge difference. God be with you.

CPSIA information can be obtained
at www.ICGtesting.com
Printed in the USA
JSHW022352160523
41821JS00003B/10